Essential Notes for Medical and Surgical Finals

KAJI SRITHARAN MBBS, BSc
Specialist Registrar in General Surgery
North West Thames, London
Honorary Research Fellow, SORA, Imperial College London

JONATHAN ROHRER MA (Cantab), MRCP
Clinical Research Fellow
Institute of Neurology

ALEXANDRA C RANKIN MBBS, BSc, MRCP
Clinical Research Fellow
King's College London

and

SACHI SIVANANTHAN MBBS, BSc (Hons)
Foundation Year Doctor
Conquest Hospital, East Sussex

Radcliffe Publishing
Oxford • New York

Radcliffe Publishing Ltd
18 Marcham Road
Abingdon
Oxon OX14 1AA
United Kingdom

www.radcliffe-oxford.com
Electronic catalogue and worldwide online ordering facility.

British Library Cataloguing in Publication Data

A catalogue record for this book is available from the British Library.

ISBN-13: 978 184619 169 5

Typeset by Pindar NZ (Egan Reid), Auckland, New Zealand
Printed and bound by TJI Digital, Padstow, Cornwall, UK

Contents

Preface

Covering both Medicine and Surgery, this is an essential revision companion for medical students and will prove to be a valuable resource for junior doctors at all stages of their training.

Examinations for undergraduate medical students and at postgraduate level can take a number of forms, including Multiple Choice and Extended Matching Questions, Single Best Answers, Short Notes, Vivas and OSCEs. This book provides the necessary information to tackle all of these exam formats successfully, and gives guidance on how to manage each topic competently in clinical practice.

The medical and surgical curricula are divided into over twenty key sections, each of which concisely cover the relevant information including definitions, aetiology, key clinical features, investigations, and management.

Comprehensive, compact and user-friendly, this book is ideal for the early stages of revision, for last minute cramming, and for use on the wards.

Kaji Sritharan
Jonathan Rohrer
Alexandra C Rankin
Sachi Sivananthan
June 2008

About the authors

Kaji Sritharan MBBS, BSc, MRCS (Eng)
Kaji trained in medicine at St Mary's Hospital Medical School and University College London, and completed her Basic Surgical Training in London. She has recently completed an MD in the field of Vascular Surgery and is currently a Specialist Registrar in General Surgery on the North West Thames Rotation. Kaji has considerable experience in teaching having held posts as an Anatomy Demonstrator and Tutor in Anatomy and Embryology at Christ Church College, University of Oxford, and as a PBL-tutor at Imperial College London, where she was also involved in organising the final MBBS Examinations.

Jonathan Rohrer MA(Cantab), MRCP
Jonathan trained at Oxford and Royal Free and University College Medical School. He has taken an active interest in medical education and teaching since qualification, including being Chairman of the Young Fellows Committee of the Royal Society of Medicine, lecturing in Neurology for finals and MRCP, and running a number of courses including Teaching Skills for junior doctors. He is currently a Clinical Research Fellow at the Institute of Neurology undertaking a PhD.

Alexandra C Rankin MBBS, BSc, MRCP
Alex trained in medicine at St Mary's Hospital Medical School, Imperial College London. After graduating from university in 2001, with triple honours and a first class honours BSc, she rotated through a variety of general medical positions, obtaining her MRCP in 2004. She commenced her training as a specialist registrar in renal medicine in January 2005. Alex takes an active interest in both undergraduate and postgraduate education. She is currently working as a Clinical Research Fellow at King's College London.

Sachi Sivananthan MBBS, BSc (Hons)
Sachi trained in medicine as a graduate entry medical student at Guy's, King's and St Thomas' (GKT) Medical School, and is currently a Foundation Year doctor at Conquest Hospital, East Sussex. She has a keen interest in teaching and was involved in trialling the peer-teaching of Anatomy at GKT medical school. She was a member on the Working Group for the International Campaign for Revitalising Academic Medicine (ICRAM) and was chairperson of the Students' group. In addition, she sits on the Council of the Clinical Section and Students' section of the Royal Society of Medicine, and has organised a number of Finals OSCE Revision Meetings.

Acknowledgements

This book would not have been possible without support and advice from the following individuals:

Dr Catherine Bagot
Dr Rupa Bessant
Mr Imad Bourghli
Dr Richard Board
Dr Kate Childs
Mr Peter Dawson
Mr Ian Franklin
Dr Clare Hooper
Dr Tricia Khoo
Dr Aliki Manoras
Dr Mark Norman
Dr Satish Jayawardene
Dr Frank Post
Dr Nadeem Rahman
Dr Gajan Rajeswaran
Mr TGV Sritharan
Mr Abbad Toma
Mr Andrew Wan
Dr Jason Warren
Dr Mark Westbrook

Medicine

Neurology

1

1.1. Neurological examination

The key to neurological diagnosis is *pattern recognition*, and there are a limited number of patterns that you need to know. Neurological examination and diagnosis is sometimes seen as difficult because emphasis is placed on lots of different individual diseases rather than patterns of disease.

Patients with weakness will fall into one (rarely two) of four syndromes representing the stages in the motor pathway from the cortex to the muscle: upper motor neurone (UMN), lower motor neurone (LMN), neuromuscular junction (NMJ), and muscle. You should be aware of the classical features for each of these syndromes.

TABLE 1.1 Patterns of Motor Disorder

	UMN	LMN	NMJ	MUSCLE
Inspection	Nil	Wasting Fasciculations	Nil	Wasting
Tone	Increased	Normal/decreased	Normal	Normal/decreased
Weakness (pattern)	Pyramidal	*See below*	Proximal (fatiguable)	Proximal
Reflexes	Increased Extensor plantars	Decreased/absent	Normal	Normal/decreased

- 'Pyramidal' weakness is the pattern seen in UMN syndromes: in the upper limb extensors are weaker than flexors; in the lower limb flexors are weaker than extensors.
- Remember that the UMN synapses with the LMN in the anterior horn of the spinal cord – this will help you remember that in motor neurone disease, a disease of the anterior horn cells, there may be both UMN and LMN signs (*although this is not the true explanation!*)
- It is useful to think of the LMN as consisting of three parts: *the root, the plexus* and *the nerve*. Patterns of weakness then depend on which part is affected. In a polyneuropathy or 'peripheral neuropathy' there is commonly distal weakness.

The two main sensory tracts are the spinothalamic tract (pain and temperature) and the dorsal columns (proprioception and vibration). Touch is carried via both. When considering patterns of sensory loss, think about the sensory pathway as it comes in from the periphery to the brain.

Patterns of sensory disorder

- Peripheral neuropathies: 'glove and stocking' distal sensory loss
- Individual nerves: sensory loss over area which nerve supplies
- Plexus or root: sensory loss over dermatome that root supplies
- Spinal cord disease – commonly produces a sensory 'level', may:
  - affect all modalities (whole cord)
  - affect vibration/proprioception only (posterior cord)
  - affect pain/temperature only (anterior cord)
  - produce dissociated loss, i.e. vibration/proprioception one limb and pain/temperature in the opposite limb (half cord, i.e. Brown-Séquard syndrome)
- Thalamus, internal capsule, sensory cortex: hemisensory loss

The other patterns to learn are those of patients with either a cerebellar syndrome or an extrapyramidal/parkinsonian syndrome who will not have true weakness or sensory disturbance. (*See* sections 11 and 14).

1.2. Epilepsy

This is the tendency to have recurrent seizures. Seizures are caused by abnormal electrical activity in the brain and can be divided into two broad groups:
- **Generalised** (Tonic-clonic, Absence, Myoclonic).
- **Partial** (Simple, Complex, Secondary generalised).

Tonic-clonic ('grand mal') seizures

Has no warning. In the tonic phase, the patient's limbs become stiff and there is loss of consciousness. Within a minute, the clonic phase starts with convulsive movements of the limbs. Breathing is irregular; there may be tongue biting and/or urinary incontinence. Following the seizure, there may be a 'post-ictal' period lasting hours where the patient feels fatigued, confused and may have a headache.

Absence ('petit mal') seizures
Mainly affects children. Occur without warning and consist of short-lived episodes of unawareness (normally lasting <30 s), during which the patient will look as though they are staring and remain still. The patient returns to normal immediately after the episode.

Complex partial seizures
Like other partial seizures these affect only part of the brain (i.e. are focal), but awareness is altered. Features of temporal lobe seizures include déjà vu, a rising sensation in the epigastrium, olfactory hallucinations, amnesia, and repetitive and stereotyped movements of the limbs or mouth.

INVESTIGATIONS
- Diagnosis relies on a good witness history. Examination is generally normal.
- Electroencephalogram (EEG) (interictal EEG is normal in ≈ 50% of cases; if EEG is repeated or sleep EEG performed only ≈ 10% will be normal) and brain CT/MRI.

MANAGEMENT
- Drug therapy: normally started after *two* clearly described unprovoked seizures. Most patients can be controlled on monotherapy:
  - *generalised tonic-clonic:* first line treatment = valproate, carbamazepine, lamotrigine
  - *partial:* first line treatment = carbamazepine, lamotrigine, valproate.

Status epilepticus
ABC, check glucose, IV access, specific management is lorazepam initially, followed by fosphenytoin or phenytoin if required. If still ongoing treat as refractory – admit to ITU, treat with an agent such as propofol. Further management is supportive.

- General advice to patients.
  - Safety measures: take care when bathing/swimming, avoid dangerous sports.
  - Driving regulations for unprovoked seizures: the patient must be advised to contact the DVLA themself; they must be seizure free for one year in order to drive; if only having seizures at night they can drive after three years.
  - Pregnancy/contraception: a higher dose of oral contraceptive pill is needed if on an enzyme-inducing drug; in addition, there is a risk of foetal malformations with older drugs (little data is available regarding the newer drugs).

1.3. Dementia
This is defined as an acquired, progressive cognitive impairment that interferes with activities of daily living. The four most common causes are Alzheimer's Disease, Vascular Dementia, Dementia with Lewy Bodies and Frontotemporal Lobar Degeneration.

1. Alzheimer's disease (AD)
Initial symptoms are usually that of memory impairment, which is episodic ('forgetting events') and/or topographical ('getting lost'). ApoE4 is a risk factor. Biochemically, acetylcholine is deficient. On MRI, there is typically bilateral

hippocampal atrophy. As the disease progresses, global cognitive impairment and global atrophy are seen. Amyloid plaques and tau-positive neurofibrillary tangles are present on post-mortem. Treatment: cholinesterase inhibitors (donepezil, rivastigmine, galantamine) do not affect the underlying disease, but roughly about ⅓ of patients will remain at the same (or slightly higher) level of function for 1–2 years.

2. Vascular dementia (VaD)
Presentation is commonly with a slowing-up of cognition or memory problems. Although the classical description is of a 'stepwise' change, there is often a slowly progressive history +/– other focal neurological signs of cerebrovascular disease. Optimisation of vascular risk factors forms the mainstay of treatment.

3. Dementia with Lewy bodies (DLB)
Main features are of parkinsonism, visual hallucinations, fluctuations in cognition and sensitivity to neuroleptics. Some patients with idiopathic Parkinson's disease will get a similar dementia later in their disease (*Parkinson's disease dementia or PDD*). Treatment: cholinesterase inhibitors may help symptoms.

4. Frontotemporal lobar degeneration (FTLD) ('*Pick's disease*')
This is a group of disorders characterised by frontal/temporal lobe atrophy, often with young onset (<65 years). There are three main syndromes:
- *frontotemporal dementia* – personality change/behavioural symptoms.
- *semantic dementia* – loss of semantic memory, i.e. conceptual knowledge.
- *progressive non-fluent aphasia* – impaired speech production.

> #### Other causes of dementia – *it is important to rule out 'reversible' causes*
> *Metabolic:* Vitamin B12/folate deficiency, hypothyroidism, Wilson's disease
> *Inflammation/infection:* HIV, multiple sclerosis, cerebral vasculitis, SLE, neurosyphilis
> *Degenerative:* Huntington's disease, progressive supranuclear palsy, CJD
> *Alcohol/toxic*
> *Structural:* chronic subdural haematoma, tumours

Creutzfeldt-Jakob disease (CJD) – *one of the diseases caused by prions*
This is rare – think of this if dementia is rapidly progressive. Onset is typically in the 60s age group in the sporadic form, but in the 20s/30s in variant CJD. In addition to dementia, there is a progressive cerebellar syndrome and myoclonus. In variant CJD there are early psychiatric (especially depression) and lower limb sensory symptoms.

1.4. Acute confusional state (delirium)
This describes a disturbance of attention, concentration and orientation (in time and place) that fluctuates throughout the day (being worse at night). Onset is over hours to days, which distinguishes it from dementia (although patients with dementia may have superimposed episodes of delirium). Patients may be either *quiet* (seemingly apathetic), or *agitated* (with motor overactivity and/or aggression).

Some causes/predisposing factors (*mnemonic A-H*)
○ Alcohol: intoxication, withdrawal, Wernicke's encephalopathy
○ Brain disorders: stroke, seizures, head injury, space-occupying lesions
○ 'Cirrhosis' (liver disease): hepatic encephalopathy
○ Drugs/overdoses/toxins: opioids, recreational drugs, steroids, anticholinergics

- ○ Electrolyte abnormalities: uraemia, hyponatraemia, hypercalcaemia
- ○ 'Fever' (infections): encephalitis, meningitis, UTI, pneumonia
- ○ Glucose: hypoglycaemia
- ○ Hypoxia

Note: often delirium is multifactorial in origin

MANAGEMENT
- Treat the underlying cause or eliminate the precipitating factor.
- Supportive measures, e.g. a quiet environment with frequent reassurance, adequate nutrition (including vitamin supplementation if necessary) and fluid resuscitation.
- Drug therapy: most patients do not require the use of drugs. However, if necessary for safety, neuroleptics (or benzodiazepines) can be used, starting at a very low dose.

1.5. The unconscious patient

Causes of reduced consciousness and coma are similar to those for delirium (*see* above). Assessment should include: monitoring of vital signs (temperature, pulse, blood pressure, respiratory rate); pupil size and reaction (dilated and unreactive in severe brainstem disease); and eye, verbal and motor responses (the Glasgow Coma Scale or GCS). Requires treatment of the underlying cause and supportive care as necessary (e.g. ITU admission).

Glasgow coma scale (GCS)

Score out of 15 and record individual scores, e.g. E4 V5 M6
- ○ Eyes open (E): 4 spontaneous, 3 to command, 2 to pain, 1 none
- ○ Verbal (V): 5 orientated, 4 confused, 3 inappropriate words, 2 incomprehensible sounds, 1 none
- ○ Motor (M): 6 obeys commands, 5 localises to pain, 4 withdraws from pain, 3 abnormal flexion to pain, 2 extension to pain, 1 none

1.6. Head injury

This is common and varies in severity from minor to life-threatening. Severity can be measured using GCS – Mild: 13–15; Moderate: 9–12; Severe: 1–8. Symptoms range from 'concussion' through to coma.

'Concussion' can be defined as a head-injury-induced change in mental function lasting less than 24 hours and associated symptoms such as headache or dizziness; should recover within a couple of weeks.

COMPLICATIONS OF HEAD INJURY
- **Skull fracture.**
- **Haemorrhage.**
  - *Extradural haematoma:* there is often a lucid interval before a decrease in consciousness; on CT, the haematoma often resembles a convex lens.
  - *Subdural haematoma:* more common than extradural haematomas; on CT, the haematoma may appear like a crescent around the side of the brain; and will be bright if acute and a similar colour to brain tissue if chronic.
  - *Subarachnoid and intracerebral haemorrhage (see below).*
- **Post-concussion syndrome:** patients often complain about symptoms (headache, dizziness, poor sleep, poor memory or concentration) many months after the initial (often mild) head injury; the cause of which is unclear.

1.7. Brain tumours

Tumours can be primary or secondary and typically present with signs of raised intracranial pressure (*see* below), seizures, or a progressively worsening focal neurological deficit.

- Primary intracranial tumours can be:
  - 'benign': grade 1 and 2 gliomas, meningiomas, pituitary adenomas and acoustic neuromas
  - 'malignant': grade 3 and 4 gliomas (grade 4 = glioblastoma multiforme).
- Secondary metastases from a carcinoma elsewhere in the body can present before signs of the primary disease.

Raised intracranial pressure (ICP)

Symptoms include: **headache** that is worse on straining, coughing, bending forwards or lying flat (e.g. worse on waking up); **vomiting**; **visual symptoms** (obscurations, i.e. transient visual loss, blurring, or double vision secondary to a sixth nerve palsy); **papilloedema** is seen on fundoscopy; if severe, there may be a **decreased level of consciousness**.

Causes
- Space occupying lesions: tumour, abscess, haematoma
- Hydrocephalus (increased CSF in the brain); classified as:
  - 'communicating' (poor absorption of CSF), e.g. after meningitis/SAH
  - 'obstructive' (CSF flow is blocked), e.g. occlusion of the ventricles by a tumour
- Oedema post-HI or infarction
- Venous sinus thrombosis
- Idiopathic intracranial hypertension

1.8. Cerebrovascular disease

Stroke

Sudden onset focal neurological deficit secondary to cerebrovascular disease, lasting >24 hours. A transient ischaemic attack (TIA) is the same, but symptoms last <24 hours. Stroke can occur secondary to:

1. **Infarction** (accounts for ≈ 3/4 of cases) due to occlusion of an artery (ischaemic stroke) by:
   - local thrombosis
   - embolism from the heart or a large artery.

   Rarely, it may be due to:
   - diseases that affect the blood (e.g. polycythaemia)
   - non-atheromatous disease of the vessel wall (e.g. dissection, vasculitis)
   - loss of perfusion ('watershed'/border-zone infarct, e.g. after cardiac arrest).

   Venous infarction (e.g. due to cerebral venous sinus thrombosis).

2. **Haemorrhage** (accounts for ≈ 1/4 of cases): intracerebral or subarachnoid.

Vascular territories affected – symptoms and signs

Anterior circulation stroke, i.e. arteries from the carotid circulation
- *Ophthalmic artery:* monocular visual loss (transient = *amaurosis fugax*)
- *Middle cerebral artery:* contralateral hemiparesis (face and upper limb > lower limb), hemisensory loss, homonymous hemianopia and neglect; aphasia if dominant hemisphere affected (e.g. Broca's or Wernicke's)
- *Anterior cerebral artery:* contralateral hemiparesis (lower limb > upper limb)

Posterior circulation stroke, i.e. arteries from the vertebro-basilar circulation
- ○ *Posterior cerebral artery:* contralateral homonymous hemianopia
- ○ *Basilar artery thrombosis:* asymmetric quadriparesis with cranial nerve signs
- ○ *Posterior inferior cerebellar artery (lateral medullary syndrome):* contralateral limb pain/temperature loss, involvement of cranial nerves 5 (ipsilateral pain/temperature loss) and 9/10 (dysarthria, dysphagia), ipsilateral Horner's syndrome, ipsilateral cerebellar signs, vestibular dysfunction (vertigo, vomiting)

Lacunar stroke, i.e. small penetrating vessels supplying white matter/basal ganglia
- ○ Contralateral hemiparesis and/or hemisensory loss with no cortical signs

INVESTIGATIONS
- All patients require CT brain or MRI scanning within 48 hours and preferably ASAP.
- Subsequent investigations for cause of stroke include ECG, Echo cardiogram and carotid duplex.

MANAGEMENT
- Medical: For infarcts, give aspirin; consider referral to specialist unit for thrombolysis if presentation is within 3 hours of onset of symptoms.
- Supportive: e.g. adequate fluids and nutrition, swallowing assessment with NG/PEG tube insertion for feeding if necessary, TEDS, monitor for infections.
- Multidisciplinary team approach: involve speech, OT, physiotherapists; consider transfer to a stroke unit as improves outcome.
- Optimise vascular risk factors: to prevent recurrence, i.e. stop smoking, treat hypertension, high cholesterol and diabetes mellitus; investigate and treat heart disease and atrial fibrillation.

Carotid dissection
Common cause of stroke in young patients and can occur spontaneously or after trauma. Patients often have ipsilateral neck pain followed by a focal neurological deficit (stroke). ≈ 50% of patients present with a Horner's syndrome.

INVESTIGATIONS AND MANAGEMENT
- Imaging: MRI normally visualises the dissection.
- Treatment: anticoagulation – initially with heparin, then warfarin.

Cerebral venous sinus thrombosis
May present with headache, seizures, focal weakness and papilloedema. Multiple risk factors – including genetic or acquired prothrombotic disorders, pregnancy, OCP, malignancy, dehydration and infection.

INVESTIGATIONS AND MANAGEMENT
- Imaging: diagnosis is confirmed by MRI +/– MRV (magnetic resonance venography).
- Treatment: anticoagulation – initially with heparin, then warfarin.

Subarachnoid haemorrhage (SAH)
Most commonly caused by rupture of an intracranial 'berry' aneurysm (≈ 85%); other causes include AV malformations.

CLINICAL FEATURES
- Sudden onset 'thunderclap' headache.
- Meningism: nausea and vomiting, stiff neck and photophobia (due to irritation of the meninges by blood).
- Altered consciousness (transient in ≈ 50%); focal neurological signs; seizures (less common – ≈ 6%).
- Complications: rebleeding, delayed cerebral ischaemia, hydrocephalus, hyponatraemia.

INVESTIGATIONS
- CT scan: >90% sensitive within 24 hours but sensitivity decreases with time.
- If CT normal but clinical suspicion exists, then lumbar puncture (LP) for xanthochromia (positive from 6–12 hours until around two weeks from onset of symptoms).
- If SAH suspected, perform cerebral angiography.

MANAGEMENT
- Supportive: including IV fluids, regular analgesia, TEDS, antiemetics and laxatives.
- Medical: nimodipine.
- Surgical: endovascular coiling (performed radiologically), or neurosurgical clipping.

1.9. Headache
Acute severe headache
This is a medical emergency. Assess GCS and for focal neurological signs, neck stiffness, rash, etc.
  Causes
- Bleeding – SAH, intracerebral haemorrhage.
- Infection – meningitis, encephalitis, systemic infections.
- Migraine.
- Intracranial pressure changes (sudden increase or decrease).
- Drugs, e.g. vasodilators.

INVESTIGATION   CT brain – most patients will then require LP.

Primary headache syndromes
Migraine
Definition: repeated episodes of throbbing pain lasting between 4 and 72 hours. Often unilateral and aggravated by movement. Associated features: nausea/vomiting, photophobia, and phonophobia. Management: treat acute episodes with simple analgesia (e.g. NSAIDs) +/– antiemetic (e.g. metoclopramide). Consider triptans if no benefit from simple analgesia. Consider prophylaxis, e.g. with propranolol or pizotifen, if there are greater than 3 episodes in one month.

Cluster headache – one of the 'trigeminal autonomic cephalgias'
Definition: episodes of severe, unilateral, orbital, supraorbital and/or temporal pain which last between 15 minutes and 3 hours and occur in clusters (1 week to 1 year), with intervening periods of at least a month. Associated features: red eye, tearing, nasal symptoms, ptosis, and miosis. Management: treat acute episodes with oxygen therapy or triptans; consider prophylaxis with verapamil or lithium.

Other primary headache syndromes

○ Tension-type headache – a 'featureless' headache, i.e. *none* of the features of migraine
○ Primary stabbing headache
○ Benign cough headache
○ Other trigeminal autonomic cephalgias, e.g. paroxysmal hemicrania

Idiopathic intracranial hypertension (IIH = new name for benign IH*)*

Most commonly affects young overweight women. Associated with OCP use and other drugs, e.g. tetracycline, vitamin A, retinoids. Clinical features: headache (due to raised ICP), visual obscurations (common) +/– blurring of vision and papilloedema on fundus examination.

Investigations: MRI to exclude a SOL or venous sinus thrombosis and LP to measure opening pressure (> 25 cmH$_2$O). Treatment: stop possible causative drugs; encourage weight loss; consider diuretics (e.g. acetazolamide); repeated LPs; if severe (e.g. if sight threatened) consider optic nerve fenestration or a CSF shunt.

1.10. Meningitis and encephalitis

Meningitis

Inflammation of the meninges normally secondary to infection but can be caused by malignancy or inflammatory disorders such as sarcoidosis. Can be *acute* or *chronic*.

Acute

Onset is over hours with acute severe headache, fever, nausea +/– vomiting, photophobia, neck stiffness and a positive Kernig's sign. In severe cases there may be confusion and decreased consciousness +/– seizures.

Infective causes of meningitis

Bacterial
○ Meningococcal (*N. meningitidis* groups B and C most common, A and W135 less common) – produces a characteristic non-blanching purpuric rash and less commonly a severe septicaemic illness with widespread rash, rapid deterioration and multi-organ failure
○ Pneumococcal (*S. pneumoniae*)
○ *Haemophilus influenzae* (more common in infants)
○ *Listeria monocytogenes* (more common in elderly)
○ Rarer causes include *S. aureus* and Gram-negative rods

Viral
○ Enteroviruses *(most cases)*
○ Herpes viruses

INVESTIGATION
● Patients with severe acute headache of unclear cause require urgent CT scanning.
● Subsequent LP with CSF analysis is the key to diagnosis (send sample to: microbiology for urgent cell count and Gram stain; virology; biochemistry for protein and glucose; for protein and glucose; and cytology – *see* CSF Analysis section below).

MANAGEMENT   Prompt empirical antibiotic treatment (usually with a third generation cephalosporin) for presumed bacterial meningitis is essential. Studies have shown concurrent treatment with dexamethasone may also be beneficial. If *Listeria* is suspected amoxicillin or ampicillin should be added in. Further treatment is supportive.

Chronic
Onset is over weeks with subacute headache; features of meningism are less common than in acute. Causes: TB, *Cryptococcus* and Lyme disease.

Encephalitis
Inflammation of the brain tissue is usually secondary to infection (usually viral). In the UK, herpes simplex (HSV) and enteroviruses are commonly implicated; worldwide other causes include Japanese B and West Nile viruses. Clinical features: fever, altered consciousness and seizures. Behaviour and cognition can be affected. Management: empirical treatment with aciclovir for presumed HSV infection.

1.11. Movement disorders
- **Akinetic-rigid syndromes** (i.e. those with bradykinesia and rigidity).
- **Dyskinesias** (abnormal involuntary movements) which can be further divided into tremor, chorea, myoclonus, tics and dystonia.

Some disorders will have >1 of these features, e.g. Parkinson's disease.

Dyskinesias
- **Tremor**: a rhythmical, alternating movement of a part of the body. Can be divided into three categories:
  - **Postural**: physiological, exaggerated physiological (causes: anxiety, sympathomimetic drugs, thyrotoxicosis, caffeine, alcohol withdrawal) or essential
  - **Rest**: Parkinson's disease (more than other akinetic-rigid syndromes)
  - **Intention**: (*increases towards end of movement as target is approached*) – cerebellar disease
- **Chorea**: brief, irregular movements that seem to flow from one part of the body to another. Causes:
  - Huntington's disease (*see* below)
  - Acanthocytosis
  - Polycythaemia vera
  - Drug-induced, e.g. neuroleptics – 'tardive dyskinesia', L-Dopa
  - Sydenham's chorea
- **Myoclonus**: sudden jerky movements; can occur in specific types of epilepsy as well as many metabolic and degenerative conditions
- **Tics**: sudden, repetitive, stereotyped complex movements that the patient can voluntarily suppress with effort, e.g. in Tourette syndrome
- **Dystonia**: sustained muscle contractions that can lead to abnormal posturing of parts of the body. Can occur as a primary condition or secondary to metabolic, neurodegenerative or structural disorders

Parkinson's disease (PD)
An 'extrapyramidal' disorder due to dopamine depletion in the basal ganglia. There is normally asymmetric onset of a triad of:
- **rest tremor** (described as 'pill-rolling' when the limb is completely relaxed)

- **bradykinesia** (a 'mask-like' face, decreased blinking, soft speech, decreased arm swing, micrographia and a slow shuffling gait)
- **'lead-pipe' rigidity** (and if tremor also present – 'cogwheel' rigidity).

Other features: loss of postural reflexes, dementia, depression, postural hypotension.

> If asked to examine for a parkinsonian disorder, you should look for the characteristic triad of features found in PD, and any other features that may suggest one of the other akinetic-rigid syndromes:
> ○ Observe the patient surroundings – is there masked facies, decreased blink rate?
> ○ Ask the patient to rest their hands on their knees and observe – is there a rest tremor?
> ○ Ask the patient to outstretch their arms – is there a postural tremor?
> ○ Ask the patient to perform fine finger movements – is there bradykinesia?
> ○ Examine the upper limb tone – is there 'lead-pipe' or cogwheel rigidity?
> ○ Examine the eye movements – is there a supranuclear gaze palsy?
> ○ Listen to the speech – does the patient have a soft, monotonous speech?
> ○ Ask the patient to write a sentence – is there micrographia?
> ○ Ask the patient to walk – is there a festinant gait with decreased arm swing and difficulty turning?
> ○ Explain that you would do a lying and standing BP (looking for postural hypotension)

MANAGEMENT
- Dopamine agonists (e.g. ropinirole or pramipexole): first line in younger patients.
- L-Dopa ('Sinemet' or 'Madopar'): first line in older patients. Important side effects include postural hypotension, hallucinations, and in long term – 'wearing off' and 'on-off' effects, dyskinesias.
- Other treatments: COMT inhibitors (e.g. entacapone), MAO inhibitors (e.g. selegiline), amantadine, deep brain stimulation.

Other akinetic-rigid ('parkinsonian') syndromes
○ Drug-induced (particularly antipsychotics)
○ 'Parkinson's plus' syndromes
  ▶ Progressive supranuclear palsy: gaze palsy, early falls, axial rigidity
  ▶ Multiple system atrophy: cerebellar, autonomic and pyramidal signs
  ▶ Corticobasal degeneration: asymmetric parkinsonism, 'alien limb' phenomenon
○ 'Vascular' parkinsonism: commonly affects lower limbs > upper limb
○ Toxins, e.g. carbon monoxide, manganese
○ Genetic conditions, e.g. Wilson's disease

Huntington's disease
This is an autosomal dominant, trinucleotide repeat disorder caused by mutations in the gene encoding for huntingtin on chromosome 4. There is 100% penetrance, anticipation in successive generations and onset is usually between 30 and 50 years. The clinical picture is variable but there is usually a triad of:
- **movement disorder** (chorea in particular but also dystonia).
- **behavioural change** (often first symptom especially depression).
- **cognitive impairment.**

MANAGEMENT Symptom control is the mainstay of treatment. There is no cure. Genetic counselling should be offered.

1.12. Speech disorders

Examination of speech disorders

At a basic level the simplest distinction you should make is between a *dysphasia (an impairment of language)* and a *dysarthria (an impairment of articulation).*

- **Listen to the patient's spontaneous speech.** The aim should be to hear enough speech to help you decide what is going on, and the best way of doing this is by getting the patient either to describe a picture or (more usefully in an exam setting) to describe the room they are sitting in. Simple questions such as 'What did you have for breakfast today?' may result in a single word answer. Furthermore, it is better to ask questions that do not rely on memory.
- As you listen, think about whether the following are normal: **articulation, fluency** (are they 'fluent' or 'non-fluent'?), **grammar** (is there agrammatism?) and whether there are any errors of speech (**paraphasias** or **neologisms**). At this point you should be able to decide if dysarthria or dysphasia is present.
- If it is a dysarthria, go on to examine:
  - **ability to repeat simple sounds** – pa, pa, pa (requires lips: seventh nerve); ta, ta, ta (requires tongue: twelfth nerve); ka, ka, ka (requires palate: tenth nerve)
  - **ability to repeat complex words** – British Constitution, West Register Street, Baby Hippopotamus. *Listen to the repeated phrase carefully – this will help you recognise the type of dysarthria (see below).*

Types of dysarthria

- ○ **Cerebellar** – slurred or staccato speech
- ○ **Bulbar** (due to LMN flaccid paralysis) – 'nasal' speech
- ○ **Pseudobulbar** (due to UMN spastic paralysis) – speech may sound indistinct, strained or 'strangled'
- ○ **Extrapyramidal** (e.g. in Parkinson's disease) – soft, slow, monotonous speech

- If it is a dysphasia, go on to examine:
  - **comprehension** – ask the patient to perform 1, 2 or 3-stage commands, e.g. take the piece of paper in your right hand, fold it in half and then put it on floor
  - **naming** of simple objects – e.g. watch, and also words of a low frequency, e.g. the parts of a watch (strap, buckle, etc)
  - **repetition** of increasing syllable length words – e.g. city, citizen, citizenship.

Types of dysphasia/aphasia and their characteristic features

Main cause is stroke, but dysphasia is also a feature of some dementias and other pathology affecting the dominant perisylvian areas:

- ○ **Broca's aphasia:** non-fluent speech, agrammatism, sound errors (phonemic paraphasias), relatively intact comprehension, problems with naming (anomia), poor repetition
- ○ **Wernicke's aphasia:** fluent speech, meaning errors (semantic paraphasias) and neologisms ('jargon') more than sound errors, impaired comprehension, anomia, poor repetition
- ○ **Conduction aphasia:** fluent spontaneous speech but particular difficulties in repeating words with phonemic paraphasias, normal grammar, intact comprehension, may have mild anomia

1.13. Multiple sclerosis (MS)

An inflammatory, demyelinating disorder of the central nervous system; 3:2

female:male ratio (in relapsing-remitting subtype); Peak incidence age 20–40 years; common in Northern Europe, North America, Australasia. There are essentially three subtypes:
- **relapsing-remitting** (in early disease 0.8–1.2 relapse per year).
- **secondary progressive** (affects 40% of relapsing-remitting subtype at 10 years).
- **primary progressive.**

PRESENTATION (MOST COMMONLY)
- Spinal cord disease, e.g. spastic paraparesis, sensory disturbance (there may be a sensory level), bladder and/or bowel problems (in 50%).
- Optic neuritis – usually unilateral (in 25%).
- Brainstem/cerebellar (affects 20%).
- Other (often later) features:
  - fatigue
  - mood changes
  - cognitive impairment
  - seizures (uncommon).
- Better prognostic signs:
  - female gender
  - early age of onset
  - onset with sensory symptoms or optic neuritis.

DIAGNOSIS   Requires evidence of at least 2 lesions within the CNS at 2 different sites at different times.

INVESTIGATIONS
- MRI (brain +/– spine) – for white matter lesions.
- Lumbar puncture – reveals oligoclonal bands in CSF but not serum.
- Evoked potentials (visual, auditory) – delayed due to conduction problem.

MANAGEMENT
- Drug therapy: high-dose steroids for acute relapses; symptomatic treatment to relieve symptoms such as:
  - spasticity, e.g. baclofen
  - bladder dysfunction, e.g. oxybutynin.
- Disease-modifying therapy, e.g. beta-interferon (for relapsing-remitting), glatiramer acetate, mitoxantrone.
- Multidisciplinary team involvement for long-term care, i.e. physiotherapy, occupational therapy and specialist MS nurse.

1.14. Cerebellar disease
Examination of cerebellar disease
If asked to examine for a cerebellar syndrome one system is as follows (DANISH):
- Observe the patient and their surroundings (wheelchair, obvious nystagmus, etc.).
- On 'finger-nose' testing – look for **I**ntention tremor and whether the finger overshoots your finger (**D**ysmetria).
- Assess alternating hand movements – is there **D**ysdiadochokinesis?
- Examine the eyes – is there **N**ystagmus?
- Listen to the speech – is the patient dysarthric with **S**taccato or **S**lurred ('scanning') speech?

● Assess **H**eel-shin co-ordination.
● Ask the patient to walk – is the patient **A**taxic (broad-based, unsteady gait)?

NB: patients rarely have the classic textbook 'H' of hypotonia.

Causes of cerebellar signs (*mnemonic is DISAPPEAR*)

○ Demyelination (MS)
○ Infarcts/haemorrhage
○ Space occupying lesions – tumours, abscesses
○ Alcohol
○ Phenytoin toxicity
○ Paraneoplastic
○ Endocrine – hypothyroidism *(rare)*
○ Ataxias – genetic, e.g. Friedreich's, spinocerebellar ataxias, ataxia telangiectasia
○ Rare metabolic causes

1.15. Dizziness

The words 'dizziness' or 'lightheadedness' can mean many things, but commonly they mean either presyncope or vertigo, the feeling of the external world moving independently (e.g. spinning or falling).

Causes of dizziness

Central
○ Brainstem disease, e.g. MS, vertebrobasilar ischaemia, basilar migraine, tumours

Peripheral
○ Benign paroxysmal positional vertigo: sudden onset, brief episodes of vertigo (normally under 30 seconds) triggered by a change of position
○ Ménière's disease: recurrent episodes, each lasting hours
○ Acute labrythinitis: lasts days to weeks

Always think of systemic disease and particularly
○ Postural hypotension
○ Cardiac arrhythmias

1.16. Cranial nerve disorders

Examination of cranial nerves

Observe the patient and their surroundings.
● **First nerve**
  ▸ Ask if there is any problem with sense of smell.
● **Eyes (second, third, fourth and sixth nerves)**
  ▸ Observation: look for ptosis, exophthalmos and ocular misalignment.
  ▸ Acuity: ask the patient if they wear glasses, then test acuity formally with a Snellen chart.
  ▸ Visual Fields: test each eye individually by confrontation bringing in a moving finger or pin from the periphery to the centre in all four quadrants.
  ▸ Pupils: assess size and shape, then check direct/consensual light reflex and accommodation reflex.
  ▸ *Explain that you would test colour vision (Ishihara plates) and examine fundi.*
  ▸ Eye movements: test pursuit movements initially, remembering to ask the patient if they have any double vision; look for nystagmus; then test saccades.

- **Fifth nerve**
  - Sensation: ask the patient to close their eyes, then assess sensation in all three divisions (ophthalmic, maxillary, mandibular), comparing each side.
  - Motor: ask the patient to clench their teeth and feel over the masseter/temporalis muscles; then ask the patient to open their mouth against resistance (note, the jaw will deviate to the side of the lesion).
  - *Explain that you would also test the corneal reflex and jaw jerk.*
- **Seventh nerve**
  - Look for facial asymmetry and wasting.
  - Ask the patient to raise their eyebrows, close their eyes tightly against resistance, show their teeth and blow out their cheeks.
- **Eighth nerve**
  - Ask the patient to repeat a number you whisper in their ear whilst the other ear is occluded with your hand.
  - If abnormal, perform Rinne's and Weber's tests using a 512Hz tuning fork.
- **Ninth/tenth nerve**
  - Ask the patient to open their mouth and say 'aah' – shine a torch in to look for symmetrical movement of the palate/uvula (note, the uvula will move away from the side of the lesion).
  - *Explain that you would check for a gag reflex and assess cough/swallowing/speech.*
- **Eleventh nerve**
  - Ask the patient to shrug their shoulders against resistance (trapezius) and turn their head to each side against resistance (feel the bulk of sternocleidomastoid with your other hand whilst examining).
- **Twelfth nerve**
  - Look at the tongue in the mouth for wasting and fasciculations.
  - Ask the patient to stick their tongue out (note, it will move towards the side of the lesion) then assess tongue movements.

Optic neuritis

This is acute inflammation of the optic nerve; *papillitis* if the nerve head is involved – when the optic disc will appear swollen; *retrobulbar neuritis* if the inflammation is behind the nerve head – when the optic disc will appear normal. Causes include: MS and viral infections.

CLINICAL FEATURES

- Decreased visual acuity, normally sudden onset and may get progressively worse over hours to days.
- Pain on movement of the eye (common).
- Central scotoma.
- Relative afferent pupillary defect.
- Impaired colour vision.
- Optic atrophy (with a pale disc) – occurs.
- Normally there is recovery of vision but some patients are left with visual loss and/or some of the clinical features above.

Visual field defects

Review anatomy of visual pathway from eye to occipital cortex; nature of field defect depends on site of pathology:
- *Retinal disease* – field defect depends on the part of retina affected, e.g. retinitis pigmentosa affects the peripheral retina causing 'tunnel vision' (i.e. constricted

peripheral fields with intact central vision), an inferior retinal vascular occlusion will lead to a superior field defect.
- *Optic nerve* – if only macular fibres are damaged there will be a central scotoma; pressure on the optic nerve mainly affects peripheral fibres, leading to tunnel vision (e.g. glaucoma, papilloedema); if the whole nerve is damaged there will be complete blindness in that eye.
- *Optic chiasm* (where nasal fibres cross) – bitemporal hemianopia.
- *Optic tract* – contralateral homonymous hemianopia.
- *Upper optic radiation (parietal)* – contralateral inferior homonymous quadrantanopia.
- *Lower optic radiation (temporal)* – contralateral superior homonymous quadrantanopia.
- *Occipital cortex* – contralateral homonymous hemianopia (often with macular sparing and therefore bilateral lesions can cause tunnel vision).

Pupillary abnormalities
Anisocoria (unequal pupil size): up to 20% of people have a 'simple' anisocoria.

Causes of miosis (small pupil)
- ○ 'Senile'
- ○ Argyll-Robertson
- ○ Pontine lesion
- ○ Opiates
- ○ Horner's syndrome
- ○ Miotic eye drops (e.g. pilocarpine)
- ○ Organophosphate poisoning

Causes of mydriasis (large pupil)
- ○ Third nerve palsy
- ○ Mydriatic eye drops (e.g. tropicamide)
- ○ Adie's pupil
- ○ Drugs (e.g. tricyclics)

Horner's syndrome is characterised by a triad of miosis, anhydrosis and ptosis. Causes: neck trauma, carotid dissection, brainstem stroke, Pancoast's tumour.

Papilloedema
Swelling of the optic discs.

Causes of papilloedema
- ○ Raised intracranial pressure (*see* above)
- ○ Accelerated hypertension
- ○ Blood disorders, e.g. severe anaemia
- ○ Drugs/toxins, e.g. lead

Eye movement disorders
When examining eye movements three questions will help establish the diagnosis:
- **Does it fit a single nerve palsy?**
  - ▸ Third nerve palsy – eye is 'down and out' with the pupil dilated and ptosis (but can be partial +/– pupil-sparing, e.g. *when associated with diabetes*).
  - ▸ Sixth nerve palsy – failure of abduction.
  - ▸ Fourth nerve palsy – double vision on downward gaze.
- **Is it an internuclear ophthalmoplegia?** Difficulty in adduction with nystagmus in the contralateral eye (*but normal convergence*); can be bilateral, due to a lesion in the medial longitudinal fasciculus (which links ocular motor nuclei in the brainstem).
- **Is it a 'complex ophthalmoplegia'**, i.e. does not fit a particular pattern? If it is

not a combination of 3, 4 and/or 6th nerve palsies then think of myasthenia gravis, thyroid eye disease, ocular myopathy. Rarely there may be a supranuclear palsy (i.e. an UMN syndrome).

Common causes of a third nerve palsy

○ Medical: diabetes (leads to nerve infarction) – pupil sparing, painless
○ Surgical: posterior communicating artery aneurysm or tumour causing compression on the nerve – pupil is affected, eye may be painful

Trigeminal neuralgia

Acute stabbing or shooting pain lasting a few seconds, which affect the maxillary or mandibular branches of the fifth nerve. Treatment: most patients controlled on drugs; first line treatment is carbamazepine.

Seventh nerve palsy

LMN palsy which affects the whole side of the face. Note: an UMN palsy spares the upper part of the face.

Causes of a LMN seventh nerve palsy

Unilateral
○ Bell's palsy (a diagnosis of exclusion), Herpes zoster ('Ramsay Hunt syndrome'), tumours (e.g. acoustic neuromas), pontine stroke

Can be bilateral
○ Sarcoidosis, Lyme disease, Guillain-Barré syndrome

Remember that myasthenia gravis or myopathies may also cause facial weakness.

This schematic diagram is a way of thinking about the causes of **cranial nerve palsies**; it describes the journey of the LMN from the cranial nerve nucleus to the 'target'.

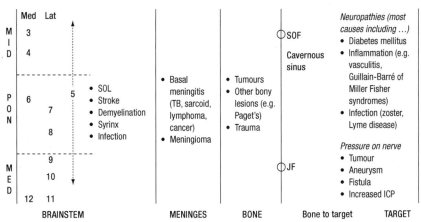

FIGURE 1.1 Causes of cranial nerve palsies.

- On the left is the brainstem, which can be divided into the midbrain, pons and medulla.
- The cranial nerve (CN) nuclei are grouped in a simple way: two above the brainstem; two in the midbrain (3, 4); four in the medulla (5–8); and four

in the pons (9–12). One proviso is that the fifth nerve nucleus is large and traverses the whole brainstem.
- The nuclei can also be grouped medially (3,4,6,12 – i.e. those you can divide into 12) and laterally.
- The nerve passes through the **brainstem**, then through the **meninges** covering the brainstem, on through the foramina in the **bone** (for example, the superior orbital fissure (SOF) and jugular foramen (JF)). Finally, each nerve takes a path from the **bone to its 'target'**, e.g. to the eye muscles for CN 3, 4 and 6. There is little clinical use in knowing these pathways in detail apart from knowing the structures which pass through the cavernous sinus.
- So, this allows us to group the causes of cranial nerve palsies anatomically, as above and allows us to see why certain nerve palsies cluster:
  - **bulbar (i.e. medulla) syndromes:** CN 5, 9, 10, 12
  - **lateral medullary syndrome:** CN 5, 9, 10
  - **cerebellopontine angle lesions:** CN 5 and 7 (and if acoustic neuroma)
  - **jugular foramen syndrome:** CN 9, 10, 11
  - **superior orbital fissure/Cavernous sinus syndromes:** CN 3, 4, 5-ophthalmic, 6 (5-maxillary can also be affected in cavernous sinus syndromes).

Never forget myasthenia gravis or myopathies as possible causes of weakness.

1.17. Disorders of the spine
Spinal cord lesions
- **Motor**
  - Spastic paraparesis or quadriparesis: an UMN syndrome causing bilateral limb weakness:
    - if thoraco-lumbar lesion – lower limbs affected only, i.e. paraparesis
    - if cervical lesion – upper and lower limbs affected, i.e. quadriparesis.
  - There may be LMN signs *at the level of the lesion only.*
- **Sensory**
  - If the whole cord, all sensory modalities will be affected below the level of the lesion (a 'sensory level').
  - In anterior lesions (e.g. anterior spinal artery infarction), pain and temperature only affected.
  - In posterior lesions (e.g. subacute combined degeneration secondary to B12 deficiency), proprioception and vibration only affected.
- **Bladder, bowel, sexual function** – variably affected in incomplete lesions.

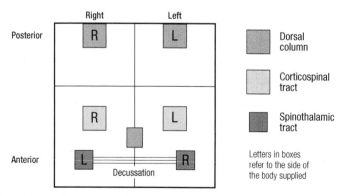

FIGURE 1.2 Schematic diagram of the cord.

Different cord syndromes

- **Whole transverse cord:** all modalities affected with a sensory 'level'; spastic paraparesis.
- **Hemisection** (i.e. Brown-Séquard syndrome): dissociated sensory loss, i.e. vibration/proprioception ipsilateral and pain/temperature contralateral; ipsilateral hemiparesis.
- **Anterior cord:** pain/temperature only affected; spastic paraparesis.
- **Posterior cord:** vibration/proprioception only affected.
- **Central** (e.g. syrinx): pain/temperature loss over levels that syrinx affects; spastic paraparesis.

Some acquired causes of a spastic paraparesis (*mnemonic is STAND*)

Not in order of frequency!
- Spondylosis of the cervical spine, Syringomyelia, Subacute combined degeneration
- Trauma
- Anterior spinal artery infarction; Abscess
- Neoplasms (primary or secondary)
- Demyelination (MS), Disc prolapse

Remember that very rarely there may be:
- a supraspinal cause, e.g. parasagittal meningioma
- an hereditary cause, e.g. hereditary spastic paraparesis (HSP)

Spinal cord compression

Acute- or subacute-onset spinal cord compression (e.g. secondary to a tumour, large disc prolapse or abscess) is a medical emergency. Management: urgent MRI and referral to surgeons are necessary.

Syringomyelia – *rare but often discussed in exams*

- Cystic cavitation in the cord
- Spastic paraparesis: seen below the level of the syrinx and LMN signs at level of the syrinx
- Sensory disturbance: as it is a central cord lesion the ascending sensory tracts themselves are often unaffected. However fibres from the spinothalamic tract are affected as they cross over to the other side, causing sensory loss of pain/temperature at the level of the syrinx only
- Can expand into brainstem ('syringobulbia') and cause associated symptoms/signs

Anterior spinal artery occlusion

- Acute onset paraparesis – may be 'spinal shock' (flaccid weakness) initially, followed by a spastic paraparesis with sensory loss below the level of the lesion with sparing of vibration/proprioception
- May be bowel/bladder sphincter involvement
- Weakness is often preceded by sudden onset of severe (radicular, i.e. root) back pain

Cauda equina syndrome

The cauda equina starts at the termination of the spinal cord.

CLINICAL FEATURES
- Low back pain +/– radiation to legs.

- LMN features: flaccid weakness, decreased/absent reflexes (pattern depends on level of lesion/roots affected).
- Saddle sensory abnormalities, poor anal sphincter tone.
- Bladder/bowel involvement, e.g. urinary retention, urinary/faecal incontinence.

The syndrome is a surgical emergency and requires urgent MRI scan of the lumbar spine and referral to surgeons for decompression.

1.18. Anterior horn cell, nerve root and plexus disease
Anterior horn cell disease
Motor neurone disease

CLINICAL FEATURES Mean age of onset 60 years but there is a large variation. Often a mix of UMN/LMN signs:
- 75% of patients start with limb symptoms.
- 25% start with bulbar symptoms (tongue wasting/fasciculations, dysphagia, dysarthria).
- ≈ 5% develop dementia (most commonly frontotemporal dementia).

MANAGEMENT No curative treatment but riluzole may prolong time to respiratory support.

Poliomyelitis
Affects the anterior horn cells – *see* ID section.

Nerve root disease (radiculopathies)
Presentation: most common symptom is pain (in lumbosacral radiculopathies patients often complain of back pain +/– 'sciatica', i.e. pain that radiates from the back down the leg). There may also be sensory +/– motor symptoms related to the nerve root(s) affected. Causes can be thought of as compressive (usually due to a herniated disc) or non-compressive.

Plexus disease (brachial/lumbosacral)
Rare and often secondary to trauma (e.g. road traffic accidents or birth injuries).
- *Brachial neuritis (neuralgic amyotrophy)* – uncertain aetiology but sometimes follows infection, vaccination, surgery or trauma. Presentation: There is severe continuous pain in the upper arm/neck radiating down the arm; 2–3 weeks later this pain subsides and weakness (+/– wasting) of muscles around the upper arm and shoulder girdle becomes apparent. There can be sensory loss over the upper arm.
- Malignant infiltration or local radiotherapy can (rarely) produce a painful brachial plexopathy.
- Lumbosacral plexopathy may occur with pelvic tumours or diabetes.

Foot drop (i.e. weakness of ankle dorsiflexion)
Presentation: a high stepping gait on the side of the foot drop. In an exam, look for presence of a foot splint. Causes can be thought of anatomically from the cortex down to the foot:

UMN lesions rarely cause only foot drop but ankle dorsiflexion is weak in any cortical or spinal cord disease affecting the corticospinal tract (i.e. when there is pyramidal weakness).

LMN
- ○ *Anterior horn cell* – motor neurone disease
- ○ *L5 nerve root* – compression secondary to a disc prolapse, tumour etc.
- ○ *Lumbosacral plexopathy*
- ○ *The individual nerve (sciatic becoming common peroneal and finally deep peroneal nerve)* – the common peroneal nerve is affected most often at the neck of the fibula by trauma or compression

Note: foot *inversion* is unaffected in peroneal nerve lesions while it is weak in L5 root lesions (and *eversion* is weak in both). In practice often difficult to tell apart.

1.19. Peripheral neuropathies (polyneuropathies)
Acute neuropathies
There are few peripheral neuropathies of acute/subacute onset. Apart from Guillain-Barré syndrome other causes are very rare (e.g. porphyria, diphtheria).

Guillain-Barré syndrome (GBS)
Presentation: acute onset reaching peak within four weeks.

CLINICAL FEATURES
- Ascending symmetrical LMN weakness.
- Sensory symptoms (although often few signs): pain can be prominent.
- Autonomic dysfunction: arrhythmias (therefore cardiac monitor), labile BP, urinary retention, constipation.

In about 70% of cases there is a preceding infection: *Campylobacter jejuni*, *Mycoplasma pneumoniae*, EBV, CMV.

INVESTIGATIONS
- Importantly – monitor respiratory function (VITAL CAPACITY – not peak flow).
- Lumbar puncture: raised protein.
- EMG: demyelinating in classical variant.

MANAGEMENT
- Supportive: regular vital capacity measurement +/– early ITU involvement, DVT prophylaxis.
- Medical: IV immunoglobulins (IVIg) – first line treatment.

Chronic neuropathies
Can be sensory or motor neuropathy alone, or sensorimotor neuropathy:
- **Motor:** distal weakness in a LMN syndrome pattern.
- **Sensory:** disturbance is classically a 'glove and stocking' sensory loss.

Some causes of *acquired* neuropathies (*mnemonic is DAMAGE*)
- ○ Diabetes mellitus, Drugs (e.g. isoniazid), Deficiencies of vitamins (e.g. B12)
- ○ Alcohol
- ○ Malignancy/Paraneoplastic; Metabolic (e.g. uraemia)
- ○ Autoimmune (Sjögren's syndrome, vasculitis); Amyloid
- ○ GBS (and its chronic form Chronic Inflammatory Demyelinating Polyneuropathy, CIDP)
- ○ Endocrine (hypothyroidism)

Remember there are many genetic causes of neuropathies, e.g. Charcot-Marie-Tooth – always ask FH!

INVESTIGATIONS
- Initial blood tests: FBC, ESR, U&Es, LFTs, glucose, protein electrophoresis, autoantibody screen, TFTs, Vitamin B12, folate.
- Nerve conduction studies/electromyography – neuropathies are either axonal (most) or demyelinating (e.g. CIDP) – *see Investigations* below.
- Nerve biopsy – indicated in a small number of patients.

1.20. Single nerve lesions (mononeuropathies)
Carpal tunnel syndrome (median nerve)
Associated with diabetes, hypothyroidism, acromegaly, RA, pregnancy. Clinical features: initially there is painful tingling at night in the hand spreading up the forearm. The patient may give a history of shaking their hand to relieve the pain. Examination: often no abnormal signs but if severe: sensory changes over palmar 3½ digits radially; weakness/wasting of the 'LOAF' muscles (particularly **A**bductor pollicis brevis but also **O**pponens pollicis, **F**lexor pollicis brevis, lateral two **L**umbricals). Phalen's and Tinel's tests may be positive but in practice are not that useful. Management: wrist splints can be helpful; surgical decompression in select cases.

Ulnar neuropathy
Damage to the ulnar nerve most commonly occurs at the elbow and less commonly at the wrist. Clinical features: sensory changes over ulnar 1½ digits (dorsal *and* palmar); may be no weakness or only weakness of the intrinsic muscles of the hand (apart from 'LOAF') +/– ulnar forearm muscles (if at elbow).

> Clues for C8/T1 radiculopathy or brachial plexopathy, rather than ulnar neuropathy, are sensory loss over inner forearm and weakness of 'LOAF'/median forearm muscles.

Common peroneal (lateral popliteal) neuropathy
The common peroneal nerve is often compressed or stretched at the head of the fibula. Clinical features: weak dorsiflexion (foot drop), foot eversion and weakness of extensor hallucis longus; variable sensory loss (often only small area over dorsum of foot), preserved ankle jerk.

1.21. Neuromuscular junction disorders
Myasthenia gravis
Clinical features: weakness that is often fatiguable – may be purely ocular (ptosis, ophthalmoplegia) or more generalised (proximal limbs +/– weakness in face or neck, dysarthria, dysphagia, dyspnoea). Investigations: diagnosis is made with EMG (decrement on repetitive stimulation) and/or positive acetylcholine receptor (AChR) antibodies. AChR antibody-negative cases may be MuSK antibody +ve. Tensilon tests are now performed less often. Mediastinal imaging (CT or MRI) for thymus enlargement/thymoma. Management: symptomatic treatment is with pyridostigmine. Immunosuppression (steroids initially then normally azathioprine). Other treatments: IVIg or plasma exchange if severe/relapse; thymectomy. Avoidance of drugs that exacerbate symptoms.

Lambert-Eaton myasthenic syndrome (LEMS)
Can be paraneoplastic (in most cases of small cell lung cancer) or sporadic. Clinical features: proximal limb weakness with autonomic features. Characteristically there are decreased/absent reflexes that return after exercise. Investigation: voltage-gated calcium channel antibodies are commonly present. Management: treat underlying cancer, and symptomatically with 3,4 diaminopyridine.

1.22. Muscle disorders

Commonly there is proximal limb weakness in muscle disease but it is important to remember that other muscles can be affected, causing facial weakness, ptosis, ophthalmoplegia, speech and swallowing problems, neck weakness and respiratory problems. The pattern of weakness may help in the diagnosis.

Causes of muscle disease

- ○ Inflammatory (e.g. polymyositis, dermatomyositis)
- ○ Drugs (e.g. steroids, alcohol)
- ○ Endocrine/metabolic (thyrotoxicosis, hypothyroidism, Cushing's, Addison's)
- ○ Mitochondrial disease
- ○ Inherited
  - ▶ Muscular dystrophies (e.g. Duchenne, Becker)
  - ▶ Myotonias (e.g. myotonic dystrophy)
  - ▶ Other congenital myopathies (lots!)

INVESTIGATIONS

- Serum creatine kinase.
- EMG ('myopathic': decreased amplitude and short duration motor unit action potentials) +/– muscle biopsy.

Polymyositis (PM)/dermatomyositis (DM)

CLINICAL FEATURES

- Proximal limb weakness which can be accompanied by pain/tenderness. Later on disease may progress to cause neck weakness, dysphagia etc.
- Rash in dermatomyositis: can present before muscle weakness; photosensitive over sun-exposed areas; heliotrope rash over eyelids; Gottron's papules (pink/red scaly lesions over knuckles).
- DM can be associated with malignancy – in adults you must investigate for this.

MANAGEMENT

- First line treatment: steroids – may be initially IV then oral.
- Second line – immunosuppressants (e.g. azathioprine) or IVIg.

Myotonic dystrophy

Autosomal dominant, trinucleotide repeat disorder, shows anticipation, onset third/fourth decade.

CLINICAL FEATURES

- Myotonia (e.g. difficulty opening hands or eyes quickly, percussion – worse in cold).
- Weakness: distally in hands, myopathic facies, bilateral ptosis, ophthalmoplegia, rarely dysarthria.
- Multisystem disease *(ABCDE)* – atrophy of the testes, balding, cataracts, cognitive impairment, cardiomyopathy, diabetes, ECG abnormalities (heart block).

INVESTIGATION   Characteristic EMG (myotonic 'dive bomber' discharges on audio).

MANAGEMENT   Supportive, genetic counselling, annual ECG/glucose dipstick/examination for cataracts, caution with general anaesthesia.

1.23. Investigations
CSF analysis

	BACTERIAL MENINGITIS	VIRAL MENINGITIS	TUBERCULOUS MENINGITIS	FUNGAL MENINGITIS	MALIGNANT
Protein	++	+	++/+++	++/+++	++
Glucose	<50% blood glucose	Normal, may be low (e.g. in mumps)	<50% blood glucose	<50% blood glucose	Normal or low
Cells	Neutro ++	Lympho	Lympho (Neutro early)	Lympho	Mixed
Other	Gram stain Culture	PCR	Z-N stain PCR Culture	India Ink Stain PCR for Cr Ag	Cytology

OTHER
* Raised protein (+ 0.4–1, ++ 1–2, +++ >2) – also seen in Guillain-Barré syndrome/CIDP (++/+++), spinal block (+++) – *note that cell count should not be raised in these conditions.*
* Oligoclonal bands (in CSF but not serum) – seen with MS, CNS vasculitis and rarely, sarcoid and syphilis.
* Xanthochromia – in SAH.

NCS/EMG

	AXONAL NEUROPATHIES	DEMYELINATING NEUROPATHIES
Amplitude	Reduced	Often normal
Conduction velocity	Usually normal	Reduced

Note: findings in neuromuscular junction and muscle disorders discussed above.

CT/MRI brain
CT is useful in acute stroke/haemorrhage, emergencies (e.g. head injury), detection of most SOLs and in the investigation of bony disease. Otherwise MRI is preferred. To distinguish between T1 and T2 images remember in T1 images grey matter (the outermost bit) appears grey; white matter (inner part of brain) appears white; and fluid is black. In T2 the opposite is true, i.e. grey matter is white, white matter is grey and fluid is white. In the commonly used FLAIR ('fluid attenuated') sequence appearances are for T2 except fluid is seen as black.

Cardiology

2.1. Ischaemic heart disease (IHD)

Stable angina: pain of cardiac origin, occurring on effort or with cold/stressful situations, relieved by rest; and stable over time. The pain is usually described as a tightness or band around the chest +/– radiates to the jaw or left arm.

Acute coronary syndromes (ACS)
- **Unstable angina**: cardiac chest pain +/– dynamic ECG changes, no enzyme rise.
- **Non ST elevation MI (NSTEMI)**: cardiac chest pain + troponin enzyme rise.
- **Myocardial infarction**: cardiac chest pain with classical ECG changes (ST elevation >2 mm in two or more chest leads, >1 mm in two or more limb leads, new left bundle branch block, dominant R waves and ST depression in V1–V3 (posterior infarction)).

Pathophysiology
- Narrowing of the coronary artery (CA) lumen by: atheromatous plaque which reduces blood flow leading to ischaemia of the myocardium; vulnerable plaques may fissure causing intra-plaque haemorrhage, thrombosis occluding the CA lumen; and vasospasm.
- Less commonly, drugs, such as cocaine, may cause spontaneous spasm of the coronary artery and cardiac pain (therefore take a careful drug history especially in the young).

Differential diagnosis of chest pain

Consider all the underlying tissues:

○ Skin	shingles
○ Musculoskeletal	trauma, costochondritis
○ Lungs	pneumonia, pulmonary embolus, pneumothorax
○ Heart	angina/ACS, pericarditis
○ Aorta	dissection
○ Oesophagus/stomach	reflux, ulcers

CLINICAL FEATURES

- Chest pain: central, crushing pain radiating to the jaw or left arm.
- Shortness of breath (SOB): indicative of pulmonary oedema (ask about orthopnoea, paroxysmal nocturnal dyspnoea (PND)).
- Collapse/dizziness: may be secondary to pain BUT may indicate a malignant arrhythmia.
- Palpitations (ask the patient to tap out the rhythm).

EXAMINATION

- Examination may be normal but look for:
  - coldness and clamminess of the peripheries
  - murmurs (may indicate ruptured chordae or septum)
  - evidence of fluid overload: ankle/sacral oedema, raised JVP, pulmonary oedema
  - tachycardia/irregular pulse (arrhythmias, e.g. atrial fibrillation (AF)).

INITIAL INVESTIGATIONS

- Blood tests: U&Es, FBC, clotting, fasting lipid profile, fasting glucose, troponin (taken at 12 hours following the onset of symptoms – indicates damage to the myocardium and used for risk stratification).
- ECG: if abnormal, patient is at increased risk of further events (risk stratification).
- CXR: for cardiomegaly and evidence of pulmonary oedema.

Risk factors for IHD

○ Hypertension	○ Diabetes mellitus
○ Hypercholesterolaemia	○ Smoking
○ Family history	○ Age and gender (males)

- ○ Others: obesity, lack of exercise, psychosocial factors (e.g. stress), chronic kidney disease, microalbuminuria, LVH, raised homocysteine level

FURTHER INVESTIGATIONS

- Exercise tolerance test (ETT) in troponin negative patients for risk stratification, only once pain has settled in the acute setting.
- Echocardiography.
- Nuclear medicine imaging.
- Coronary angiography.

MANAGEMENT

Initial is, as always, ABC, and appropriate treatment for ACS/MI (*see* below); further:

- **risk factor modification:** smoking cessation, tight control of blood glucose and BP, cholesterol control, exercise and weight loss if obese
- **symptom control:** nitrates, calcium channel blockers, β-blockers, nicorandil

- to improve prognosis: aspirin, clopidogrel, β-blockers, statins for cholesterol, ACE-inhibitor if LVF, spironolactone if LVF
- invasive intervention: coronary angioplasty +/– stenting (PCI), coronary artery bypass grafting (CABG).

MANAGEMENT OF MYOCARDIAL INFARCTION/ACUTE CORONARY SYNDROME
- Oxygen therapy (high flow).
- Cardiac monitor.
- Aspirin (300 mg) and stat dose 300 mg clopidogrel (also in NSTEMI).
- GTN (sublingual then IV if chest pain continues).
- IV morphine 5–10 mg IV (and metoclopramide 10 mg IV).
- Low molecular weight heparin if ACS or thrombolysis with tPA if MI.
- Consider β-blocker +/– ACE-inhibitor if safe to do so.
- Consider primary percutaneous coronary intervention (PCI) if available for MI.

Contraindications to thrombolysis

○ Absolute: previous haemorrhagic cerebrovascular accident (CVA), other CVA within last 6 months, active bleeding, suspected dissection
○ Relative: uncontrolled BP, oral anticoagulants, INR > 2.5, known bleeding disorder, recent trauma/surgery, pregnancy, traumatic CPR, active ulcers/internal bleeding (<4 weeks)

Complications of MI

Arrhythmias	Ventricular aneurysm
Heart failure	Heart defects (VSD or ruptured papillary muscle)
Dressler's syndrome	Embolic disease
Cardiac tamponade	Death

2.2. Heart failure (HF)

A pathophysiological state in which the heart cannot pump adequate supplies of blood to oxygenate the organs of the body. Low output HF is caused by the heart not functioning adequately; while in high output HF the heart is normal but the body has increased requirements.

Causes of left ventricular failure (LVF)

○ IHD, hypertension, valvular disease (MR/AR/AS), ventricular septal defect, cardiomyopathies, arrhythmias

Causes of right ventricular failure (RVF)

○ Usually 2° to LVF, but other causes include valvular disease (PR/TR/PS), cardiomyopathies, lung disease, e.g. pulmonary embolus/pulmonary hypertension

High output failure

○ Anaemia, thyrotoxicosis, systemic arteriovenous (AV) fistulae, thiamine deficiency, skeletal diseases, e.g. Paget's disease

CLINICAL FEATURES
- LVF: shortness of breath (SOB), cough with frothy, pink sputum, PND/orthopnoea. On examination, raised respiratory rate, displaced apex beat, bi-basal fine crepitations, third heart sound.
- RVF: raised JVP, swelling of ankles (SOA), sacral oedema, hepatomegaly, ascites.

INVESTIGATIONS   (*Note*: it is crucial to investigate the cause of the HF)
- Blood tests: U&Es, FBC, LFTs, clotting (for coagulopathy due to hepatic congestion), troponin, fasting cholesterol, fasting glucose.
- ECG: for ischaemia, arrhythmias, LVH.
- CXR: for cardiomegaly, upper lobe blood diversion, Kerley B lines, pleural effusions.
- Echocardiography: for degree of ventricular dysfunction, valvular lesions, VSD.
- Coronary angiography: for underlying ischaemia.

MANAGEMENT
- Should involve a multidisciplinary team approach, including heart failure specialist nurses to initiate a cardiac rehabilitation program.
- Treat the cause: e.g. if due to IHD – risk factor modification and PCI or CABG; if due to valvular disease – consider valve replacement.
- Treatment of the symptoms:
  - lifestyle modification: weight loss if obese, fluid/salt restriction
  - diuretics, e.g. furosemide
  - cardiac rehabilitation improves exercise tolerance and quality of life
  - avoidance of exacerbating factors, e.g. NSAIDs.
- Treatment to improve prognosis:
  - ACE-inhibitors, Angiotensin receptor blockers
  - β-blockers (not in acute heart failure)
  - spironolactone
  - consider aspirin/statin in IHD
  - hydralazine/nitrates in black population.
- Consider anticoagulation if patient is in AF, heart is very dilated or evidence of thromboembolic disease.
- Surgically, cardiac resynchronisation therapy with biventricular pacemakers may improve survival in select cases, and cardiac transplantation has been shown to improve both quality of life and survival. LVADs can be a bridge to transplantation.

Management of acute pulmonary oedema

Requires swift action as hypoxia can be life-threatening.
- Sit patient up and give high flow oxygen via a face mask
- GTN sublingually followed by IV infusion 2–10 mg/hr (keep systolic BP>100)
- Diamorphine 2.5 mg IV or morphine 5 mg IV + metoclopramide 10 mg IV
- Furosemide IV 40–80 mg

2.3. Hypertension (HT)

Categorised as **essential hypertension**, i.e. no cause identified, or **secondary hypertension**, i.e. hypertension due to an identifiable pathological cause, such as:
- renal disease: renal artery stenosis (RAS).
- endocrine: phaeochromocytoma, Conn's syndrome, Cushing's syndrome
- coarctation of the aorta
- drugs, e.g. NSAIDs/steroids.

British Hypertension Society classification of HT

Grade 1 (mild):	140–159/90–99
Grade 2 (moderate):	160–179/100–109
Grade 3 (severe):	above 180/110

Once HT is identified, a careful history and examination should be taken to establish:
- an identifiable cause
- associated cardiovascular risk factors
- evidence of end organ damage (e.g. retinal examination, urine dipstick for blood/protein).

INVESTIGATIONS
- Blood tests: serum creatinine and electrolytes, fasting serum glucose, fasting lipid profile.
- ECG (for left ventricular hypertrophy).
- Relevant tests for secondary causes of HT, e.g. urinary catecholamines, urinary cortisol, dexamethasone suppression test, MRA for RAS.

Who to treat?

British Hypertension Society (BHS) Guidelines suggest treatment for all patients with sustained Grade 2 HT (>160/100) and treatment of patients with Grade 1 HT (>140/90) if there is evidence of cardiovascular disease or other target organ damage, or diabetes, or if the 10-year risk of developing CV disease is >20%

What to aim for?
Target BP <140/85, unless patient has cardiovascular disease, chronic kidney disease or diabetes, in which case aim for a BP <130/80.

MANAGEMENT
- Lifestyle changes: weight loss, regular exercise, reduction of salt and fat intake, smoking cessation.
- Drug therapy: if <55 years, ACE-inhibitors are first line; if >55 years, calcium channel blockers or diuretics are first line. If a step up from monotherapy is required, consider combinations of ACE-inhibitors, calcium channel blockers and diuretics. *Note*: β-blockers not recommended (as diabetogenic).
- Other treatment:
  - for secondary prevention, all patients should be prescribed aspirin and a statin
  - for primary prevention, selected patients at higher risk should be prescribed aspirin and a statin (e.g. those with a >20% 10-year risk of developing cardiovascular disease).

2.4. Cardiac arrhythmias
Tachycardias = heart rate (HR) >100 bpm
Sinus tachycardia
Common in sick patients and can be due to a number of causes.

Atrial fibrillation (AF)
Multiple areas within the atria discharge, causing the atria to 'fibrillate'– no P waves seen on ECG.

Causes of AF

- Cardiac: IHD, rheumatic heart disease, cardiomyopathy, pericarditis, Wolff-Parkinson-White (WPW) syndrome, atrial septal defect (ASD)
- Lone AF (no cause found)
- Endocrine: thyrotoxicosis

- ○ Respiratory: pneumonia, pulmonary embolus (PE), lung cancer
- ○ Excess alcohol

INVESTIGATIONS
- ● ECG to confirm diagnosis.
- ● Tests to establish cause: troponin (?IHD); CXR (?pneumonia); TFTs; check K^+ and Mg^{2+}; consider electrophysiological studies.

MANAGEMENT
- ● Treat underlying cause: correct electrolyte abnormalities; control rate or cardiovert. Ablation up to 80% successful (typically 60%).

  High risk patients are those with HR>150 and/or critical perfusion
  - ○ Urgent treatment with heparin + synchronised DC cardioversion
  - ○ If fails, amiodarone 300 mg IV over one hour, attempt DC cardioversion again if necessary

  Intermediate risk patients are those with HR 100–150, often with symptoms of SOB
  - ○ Onset <24 hrs, unstable: then treat as for high risk
  - ○ Onset >24 hrs, unstable: heparin/warfarin + amiodarone, cardiovert later if indicated*
  - ○ Onset <24 hrs, stable: heparin + amiodarone or cardioversion
  - ○ Onset >24 hrs, stable: heparin/warfarin and rate control with β-blockers, verapamil, diltiazem, digoxin. Cardiovert later if indicated*

  Low risk patients are those with HR<100, well
  - ○ Onset <24 hrs heparin + amiodarone, cardioversion
  - ○ Onset >24 hrs heparin/warfarin, cardiovert later if indicated*

  *If onset of AF >24 hours then risk of embolisation, therefore give heparin then warfarin for one month prior to cardioversion

If you suspect fast AF in WPW, beware of medications slowing conduction via AV node as these will *increase* conduction via the accessory pathway.

Atrial flutter
Different mechanism to AF: fast circuit in right atrium. Atrial rate is 300 beats/min (sawtooth P waves seen on ECG) but block at theAV node is usual (commonly 2:1 block, 150 bpm). Causes are the same as for AF. Treatment: requires either breaking the circuit with drugs acting on atria (e.g. flecainide) or cardioversion, or blocking conduction through the AV node with drugs such as verapamil, diltiazem, or a β-blocker. Ablation is also effective, offering 95% cure. Anticoagulation is necessary.

Supraventricular tachycardias
Conduction is either via a fast pathway through the AV node, or via an accessory pathway as in WPW syndrome. Treatment: oxygen (high flow); vagal manoeuvres; then proceed to adenosine (beware may exacerbate bronchospasm in asthmatics and effect is increased by dipryridamotle: initially 6 mg, then 12 mg/12 mg/12 mg). If no response, consider drugs which act on the AV node (except in WPW), or if unstable, synchronised DC cardioversion.

Broad complex tachycardias
See Emergencies section below.

Bradycardias HR<60

Sinus bradycardia

Aetiology: seen in young, fit people; with drugs, e.g. β-blockers; and also hypo-thermia, hypothyroidism, raised intracranial pressure. If symptomatic, assess for an underlying reversible cause and treat; consider permanent pacemaker (PPM) if no treatable cause found.

Sinus node disease/sick sinus syndrome

Aetiology: caused by fibrosis around the sino-atrial (SA) node causing pauses and tachycardias (tachy/brady syndrome). Treat with insertion of PPM.

Heart block

- **First degree:** prolongation of PR interval; treatment not required.
- **Second degree:**
  - Mobitz Type 1: PR interval increases gradually leading to a dropped QRS complex
  - Mobitz Type 2: P wave occurs with no conduction to the ventricle in a 2:1, 3:1, etc. fashion. Pacing indicated.
- **Third degree heart block/complete heart block (CHB):** complete dissociation between P waves and QRS complexes – PPM indicated.

If adverse signs present (BP<90, HR<40, ventricular arrhythmias, HF) *or* risk of asystole (recent asytole, Mobitz Type 2, CHB, ventricular pauses >3 secs) then urgent treatment is necessary: atropine 500 mcg IV (max 3 mg), consider adrenaline and temporary pacing.

2.5. Valvular heart disease

CLINICAL FEATURES

- Systolic murmurs are graded 1–6 depending on severity; diastolic murmurs are graded 1–4.
- Left-sided murmurs are louder in expiration, whereas right-sided murmurs are louder in inspiration.
- Loudness of the murmur does not necessarily correlate with severity.
- Ejection systolic murmur (ESM)   AS   PS   ASD   HOCM
- Pansystolic murmur (PSM)   MR   TR   VSD

	AORTIC STENOSIS	AORTIC REGURGITATION	MITRAL STENOSIS	MITRAL REGURGITATION
Causes	Rheumatic fever	Rheumatic fever	Rheumatic fever	Rheumatic fever
	Bicuspid valve	IE	Rare causes:	IHD
	Calcified valve	Aortic dissection	Calcified valve	Mitral valve prolapse
	Congenital	Syphilis	Rheumatoid arthritis	Dilated LV (functional MR)
		Connective tissue diseases (CTD) e.g. Marfan's, Ank. Spond.	SLE	CTD
		HT	Carcinoid	IE or papillary muscle rupture

(continued)

	AORTIC STENOSIS	AORTIC REGURGITATION	MITRAL STENOSIS	MITRAL REGURGITATION
Symptoms	Angina LOC SOB Sudden death	Symptoms of LVF	Symptoms of LVF Haemoptysis	Symptoms of LVF
Murmur Systolic (SM) Diastolic (DM)	ESM in aortic area radiating to neck	Early, high-pitched DM at left sternal edge (louder in exp. Sitting forward)	Low-pitched mid-DM (louder in L lateral position on expiration)	PSM at apex radiating to axilla
Heart sounds	Second HS soft		Loud first HS Opening snap	Soft first HS, third HS
Pulse	Slow rising	Collapsing	May be in AF	
Apex	Heaving	Displaced, thrusting	Tapping	Displaced, thrusting
LVF	+	+	−	+
**Pulmonary HT	−	−	+	+
Investigations	ECG: LVH, LBBB CXR, Echo	ECG: LVH CXR, Echo	ECG: AF, P mitrale CXR, Echo	ECG: P mitrale CXR, Echo
Treatment	**Surgery** in symptomatic or those with gradient >50 mmHg, valve area <1 cm²	**Medical**: reduce afterload (e.g. diuretic, ACE-inhibitor) **Surgery** if evidence of LVF	**Medical** if not severe (treat HF and AF) **Surgery** if pulm. HT, symptoms significant	**Medical** if symptoms mild **Surgery** if significant symptoms or LVF

**Signs of pulmonary HT: right ventricular heave, raised JVP, loud P2, ascites, oedema.

Prosthetic valves can be metallic or tissue; metallic first HS = mitral valve replacement; metallic second HS = aortic valve replacement. Warfarinisation is required for metallic valves. Complications: endocarditis, thromboembolic disease, and haemolysis.

2.6. Infective endocarditis (IE)

Fifty per cent involve a previously normal valve, but increased risk if abnormal valve.

CLINICAL FEATURES
- Fever, night sweats, lethargy, weight loss.
- New/changing murmurs, heart failure (if valve destroyed), or heart block.
- Features of vasculitis: rash, splinter haemorrhages, Janeway lesions, Osler's nodes, Roth's spots.
- Embolisation of vegetation leading to metastatic abscesses (e.g. stroke).
- May be a recent history of dental extraction (*S. 'viridans'*), pelvic surgery (*Enterococcus*) or IV drug abuser (*Staph.* – affects right-sided valves).

INVESTIGATIONS
- >3 blood cultures: must be taken from 2 different sites at 2 different times.

- ECG: PR interval prolonged if aortic root abscess – monitor daily.
- CXR: for septic pulmonary emboli in right sided IE, heart failure.
- Echocardiography: transoesophaegeal echocardiography is most sensitive for diagnosis of vegetations.
- Blood tests: normocytic anaemia, raised inflammatory markers (e.g. CRP, ESR), renal failure, low C3/C4.

Common organisms

- ○ *Streptococcus 'viridans'* (50%)
- ○ *Enterococcus faecalis*
- ○ *Staphylococcus aureus*
- ○ HACEK organisms (*Haemophilus, Actinobacillus, Cardiobacterium, Eikenella, Kingella*)
- ○ Rarely fungal
- ○ Remember non-infective causes (malignancy, Libman-Sacks, i.e. SLE)

MANAGEMENT

- Antibiotics: IV flucloxacillin and gentamicin should be started if IE suspected. Further treatment depends on the organism but in general treat for at least four weeks (or six if prosthetic valve):
  - ▹ *Staph.* Sp: flucloxacillin
  - ▹ *Strep.* Sp: benzylpenicillin (+/– gentamicin)
  - ▹ *Enterococcus.* Sp: amoxicillin + gentamicin
  - ▹ HACEK organisms: amoxicillin (+ gentamicin for two weeks).
- Monitor response to antibiotic therapy with serial CRP measurements.
- Surgery: consider if heart failure, persistent infection, embolisation.
- Prophylaxis: consider prophylaxis in at-risk patients receiving dental, upper respiratory tract, genito-urinary, obstetric/gynaecological or GI procedures.

Rheumatic fever

Precipitated by group A Streptococcal infection. Diagnosis: based on evidence of *Strep.* infection (positive throat swab, raised serum anti-streptolysin titre, etc) and on the Revised Jones Criteria which require 2 major, or 1 major + 2 minor criteria to be present for diagnosis.

- ○ *Major criteria:* carditis, polyarthritis, subcutaneous nodules, erythema marginatum, Sydenham's chorea
- ○ *Minor criteria:* fever, arthralgia, previous rheumatic fever or rheumatic heart disease

Treatment: NSAIDs, management of heart failure, a course of penicillin followed by prophylactic antibiotics (time-scale for prophylaxis not well defined).

2.7. Cardiomyopathies and pericardial disease

Cardiomyopathies

- **Dilated cardiomyopathy (enlarged heart)** Causes: familial (25%); clinical features include biventricular failure, function MR/TR. Management: as for HF, IHD, HT, alcohol, connective tissue disease, haemochromatosis, cytotoxies may produce similar clinical features.
- **Hypertrophic obstructive cardiomyopathy (thickened heart muscle)** Cause: inherited (seek family history of sudden death). Clinical features: similar to aortic stenosis. Hypertrophic septum on echo. Management: β-blockers (if chest pain, SOB), amiodarone (for arrhythmias), consider myectomy and PPM.

- **Restrictive cardiomyopathy (stiff heart muscle)** Causes: amyloid, carcinoid, idiopathic fibrosis.
- **Arrhythmogenic right ventricular cardiomyopathy:** fatty replacement of the heart muscle leading to ventricular arrhythmias and sudden death.

Acute myocarditis
Inflammation of the myocardium. Causes: viral (Coxsackie), Lyme disease, diphtheria, rheumatic fever, radiotherapy/drugs. Clinical features: fever, chest pain, dyspnoea, dizziness, heart failure, raised CK. Management: supportively, bedrest. Complications: pericardial effusion.

Pericarditis
Causes: viruses (Coxsackie), TB (calcification on CXR), malignancy, Dressler's syndrome, radiotherapy, connective tissue disease (e.g. SLE), uraemia. Clinical features: classically, sharp, pleuritic, central chest pain, relieved by leaning forward. Listen for a pericardial rub. Investigations: widespread ST elevation on ECG except in lead aVR. Management: treat underlying cause, NSAIDs; steroids if resistant. Complications: pericardial effusion, cardiac tamponade.

Constrictive pericarditis
Causes: TB, intrapericardial haemorrhage from cardiac surgery, idiopathic or may follow any episode of pericarditis. Clinical features: severe RVF can occur. Investigations: CT shows pericardial thickening + calcification. Treatment: consider surgical excision of pericardium.

Pericardial effusion/tamponade
Causes: may follow any cause of pericarditis or secondary to trauma. Clinical features: tamponade is associated with a raised JVP which rises further on inspiration (Kussmaul's sign), hypotension which drops further on inspiration (pulsus paradoxus), quiet heart sounds. Investigations: CXR reveals a large globular heart; ECG shows low voltage complexes. Echo confirms the presence of an effusion. Management: tamponade is a medical emergency and requires immediate drainage of the effusion (needle pericardiocentesis).

2.8. Congenital heart disease
Acyanotic congenital heart disease
Atrial septal defect
Ostium secundum defects are more common and are high in the atrial septum; septum primum defects are lower and typically affect the AV node leading to conduction problems. Clinical features: in adults symptoms relate to onset of atrial fibrillation and heart failure; may rarely present with CVA (paradoxical embolus). An ESM is heard over the pulmonary area and there is wide, fixed splitting of the second heart sound. ECG reveals RBBB with right axis deviation (secundum) or left axis deviation (primum). Management: involves closure of the defect. Complications include: Eisenmenger's syndrome.

Ventricular septal defect (VSD)
Aetiology: may be congenital, associated with Down's syndrome or can complicate myocardial infarction. Clinical features: may present with heart failure, a pansystolic murmur is heard on examination. Treatment: involves closure of the defect. Complications: arrhythmias (atrial fibrillation, ventricular tachycardia), infective endocarditis, Eisenmenger's syndrome.

Patent ductus arteriosus (PDA)

The ductus arteriosus connects the pulmonary artery to the aorta in the foetus and closes at birth. PDA occurs if the vessel does not close. Presentation: heart failure, infective endocarditis, pulmonary hypertension may occur. Investigations: diagnosis is by echocardiography. Management: consider either indomethacin, percutaneous closure or surgery.

Coarctation of the aorta

Narrowing of the thoracic aorta distal (usually) to the left subclavian artery. Clinical features: presentation may be with hypertension, low BP and diminished lower limb pulses. Management: consider stenting or surgical repair.

Cyanotic congenital heart disease
Fallot's tetralogy

A combination of pulmonary stenosis (PS), VSD, overriding aorta, right ventricular hypertrophy (RVH). Presentation: with cyanosis in the newborn (hypercyanotic spells due to RV outflow obstruction), or later in life following incidental detection of the murmur, or heart failure. Management: involves surgical correction. A Blalock shunt connecting the aorta with the pulmonary artery may be life-saving and buy time for further surgery.

Transposition of the great arteries

The aorta arises from the right ventricle and the pulmonary artery from the left ventricle. Survival depends on the two circulations mixing. Treatment: surgical correction is required.

2.9. Emergencies
Cardiac arrest

- In the unresponsive patient assess airway, breathing and circulation (ABC).
- Confirm cardiac arrest.
- CALL RESUSCITATION TEAM.
- Initiate cardio-pulmonary resuscitation (CPR); 30 compressions to two breaths, while attaching cardiac monitor to the patient.
- Once monitor applied assess rhythm on monitor.
- If shockable rhythm (ventricular fibrillation (VF) or pulseless ventricular tachycardia (VT)) then:
  - give one shock 150–360 J biphasic or 360 J monophasic
  - immediately resume CPR 30:2 for two minutes, then reassess rhythm
  - shock once more if shockable rhythm persists
  - continue the above cycle with CPR and cardioversion until rhythm change.
- If non-shockable rhythm (pulseless electrical activity (PEA)/asystole):
  - resume CPR 30:2 for two minutes
  - reassess rhythm
  - if no change in rhythm and patient remains pulseless continue CPR for two minutes, then reassess rhythm, and continue cycle as necessary.

While performing CPR:
- correct reversible causes
- secure intravenous access, take urgent bloods, perform an arterial blood gas to assess oxygenation, acidosis, and check K^+
- secure airway and give oxygen (anaesthetist on arrest team)
- once airway is secure, continuous compressions is advised
- consider drugs: adrenaline 1 mg IV every 3–5 mins, amiodarone (if shockable

rhythm), atropine 3 mg (if asystole/slow PEA), sodium bicarbonate (if acidotic), calcium gluconate (if K+ high).

If PEA arrest consider 4 H's (hypoxia, hypovolaemia, hypo/hyperkalaemia, hypothermia) and the 4 T's (tamponade, thromboembolism, tension pneumothorax, toxins/therapies).

Cardiogenic shock
Associated with a high mortality rate. Occurs when the heart cannot maintain a circulation. Causes: myocardial infarction, arrhythmia, aortic dissection, tamponade, IE/valvular problem, pulmonary embolism, tension pneumothorax. Management: admit to a coronary care unit, reverse obvious cause, support circulation with inotropes, consider intra-arterial balloon pump insertion.

2.10. Cardiac investigations and interventions
Exercise tolerance test (ETT)
Indications: a diagnostic tool for patients with chest pain of intermediate risk and a prognostic tool in patients with known ischemic heart disease. Limitations: low sensitivity and specificity; not all patients', e.g. immobile patients, etc. able to perform test. Bruce protocol uses a treadmill with graded levels of exercise, with BP and ECG monitoring. Modified Bruce protocol is used after an episode of acute coronary syndrome/myocardial infarction. Contraindications: acute MI, ACS, uncontrolled arrhythmias, severe AS, symptomatic HF, active endocarditis/myocarditis/pericarditis, aortic dissection. Positive test if BP drops, chest pain, or >2 mm ST depression.

24 hour blood pressure cuff
Indications: for variable BPs in clinic, to rule out the 'white coat effect'; to evaluate resistant hypertension/nocturnal HT; to assess efficacy of drug treatment.

24 hour ECG
Indications: to assess patients with symptoms suggestive of arrhythmia (e.g. palpitations, syncope) if unable to capture with normal ECG.

Echocardiography/nuclear medicine
- **Transthoracic echocardiogram:** evaluates structure of the heart, valves, and used to assess function of the left and right ventricles.
- **Transoesophageal echocardiogram** (TOE): used to gain better images of the heart and its valves, e.g. to study the valves more closely in infective endocarditis.
- **Stress echocardiogram:** uses similar to ETT, i.e. to diagnose and prognosticate coronary artery disease. Stress is induced by exercise or with drugs, e.g. dobutamine.
- **Thallium scan:** similar indications as ETT/stress echocardiography.
- **MUGA scan:** used to evaluate LV function.

Percutaneous coronary intervention (PCI) vs Coronary artery bypass grafting (CABG)
Current studies suggest that PCI produces similar results to CABG, except in diabetics who do better with CABG. Indications: consider CABG in patients with multi-vessel disease, with left main stem disease, and in diabetics.

3

Respiratory disease

3.1. Upper respiratory tract disease

Common cold
Viral in origin (rhinovirus). Clinical features: headache, fever, blocked/runny nose. Self-limiting.

Pharyngitis (sore throat)
Usually caused by an adenovirus. Self-limiting.

Sinusitis/tonsillitis
See ENT section

Influenza virus types A and B
Type A – is responsible for pandemics due to antigenic shift (haemagglutinin antigen and neuraminidase antigen mutate so that humans immune to one strain of virus are susceptible to other strains).

CLINICAL FEATURES   Fever, cough, headache, sore throat, muscle aches. May be complicated by secondary bacterial infection (*if Staph.* species then mortality high).

DIAGNOSIS   Serological testing (not usually necessary).

MANAGEMENT   Treatment is supportive (antibiotics if secondary bacterial infection).

PREVENTION   Vaccination of susceptible individuals, e.g. patients with chronic renal failure, chronic heart and lung disease, diabetes mellitus and the elderly.

Acute stridor

This is a medical emergency. Partial upper airways obstruction causes noise on inspiration. Causes: as for any obstruction, the cause is either in the lumen, in the wall of the tube, or extrinsic to the tube:
- in the airway: foreign body, aspiration
- in the wall: tumour, oedema/spasm (allergy, infection, burns).
- outside the airway: goitre, lymph nodes.

MANAGEMENT
- Invole ENT/anaesthetics.
- Give oxygen and nebulised adrenaline.
- Consider intubation or cricothyroidotomy if risk of losing airway.
- Ultimately, treat cause (e.g. antibiotics for infection, removal of foreign body).

3.2. Shortness of breath

Causes of SOB

Lung disease
- Chest infection/pneumonia
- Lung cancer
- Pulmonary embolism
- Pulmonary fibrosis
- Asthma/COPD
- Pleural effusion
- Pneumothorax

Other
- Left ventricular failure
- Anaemia
- Foreign body inhalation
- Chest wall deformity
- Metabolic acidosis

3.3. Chronic obstructive pulmonary disease (COPD)

COPD is a term for chronic airways disease that includes chronic bronchitis and emphysema, disorders which overlap:
- **Chronic bronchitis** is defined *clinically* as: cough productive of sputum, on most days, for three months, for two consecutive years; caused by smoking.
- **Emphysema** is defined *pathologically* by: permanent dilation of the airways distal to the terminal bronchioles. Causes: smoking, rarely α-1-antitrypsin deficiency (suspect in the young with co-existing liver disease).

DIAGNOSIS   Based on history, examination, and confirmation of non-reversible airflow obstruction on spirometry (FEV1 <80% of predicted, FEV1/FVC 0.7).

CLINICAL FEATURES
- SOB on exertion, wheeze, and chronic cough with sputum production.
- Important questions to ask in the history:
  - exercise tolerance: how far can they walk, when well versus unwell?
  - sputum: increase in amount or change in colour?
  - current therapy: are they prescribed home nebulisers or oxygen?
  - are they still smoking?
- Examination: may reveal cyanosis, hyperinflated chest, reduced distance between the sternal notch and thyroid cartilage, prolonged expiration,

raised respiratory rate (RR), reduced breath sounds, wheeze and evidence of pulmonary HT.

INVESTIGATIONS
- FBC: polycythaemia.
- ABG: type 1 or 2 respiratory failure.
- CXR: hyperexpanded lungs.
- Spirometry: airflow obstruction.
- Sputum microscopy and culture.
- ECG: AF, P-pulmonale.

MANAGEMENT OF STABLE COPD – MULTIDISCIPLINARY APPROACH
- Smoking cessation.
- Pulmonary rehabilitation.
- Dietetic advice if BMI high or low.
- Pneumococcal/influenza vaccinations.
- Pharmacological management:
  - initially short-acting β-agonist and/or anticholinergic bronchodilators; if no better or ≥2 exacerbations/year consider long-acting bronchodilators
  - if no better or FEV1<50% predicted or ≥2 exacerbations/year consider inhaled steroids
  - still no better, consider oral theophyllines
  - trial of home nebulisers if symptoms distressing or disabling (although no evidence to suggest they prevent hospital admissions or improve quality of life).
- Long-term oxygen therapy for 15 hours/day if pO_2<7.3 kPa, or pO_2 7.3–8 kPa and secondary polycythaemia, nocturnal hypoxaemia, pulmonary hypertension.
- Surgical: lung volume reduction surgery, bullectomy, lung transplantation.

MANAGEMENT OF ACUTE EXACERBATIONS OF COPD
- Oxygen to keep sats >90% but <95% (watch for CO_2 retention).
- Salbutamol/ipratropium nebulisers.
- Short course of oral steroids.
- Antibiotics if sputum purulent or other evidence of infection.
- Consider non-invasive ventilation: indicated in hypoxia with raised pCO_2 and respiratory acidosis.
- Consider ITU if appropriate.
- Adequate discharge planning.
- Involve respiratory nurse.
- Consider other diagnoses such as pulmonary embolus or pneumothorax.

3.4. Asthma
1000–2000 deaths per year occur in the UK from acute asthma; in addition, produces significant morbidity. Reversible airflow obstruction due to bronchiolar smooth muscle contraction, mucus plugging, and mucosal inflammation/oedema.

CLINICAL FEATURES
- Important features in the history:
  - nocturnal cough: does the patient have disturbed sleep?
  - diurnal variation (morning dip)
  - wheeze, SOB

‣ atopy: eczema, allergies, hayfever
‣ precipitants: cold, exercise, infection, acid reflux
‣ number of days off work
‣ if it is worse during week, could it be occupational asthma?
‣ current treatment, previous hospital visits
‣ if patient has been to ITU before, suggests more severe asthma.
● Signs: polyphonic wheeze, raised respiratory rate and heart rate, cyanosis.

INVESTIGATIONS
● Peak Expiratory Flow Rate (PEFR).
● Spirometry.
● CXR (to rule out pneumothorax).
● ABG.

MANAGEMENT   British Thoracic Society 5-step guidelines:
● Step 1: inhaled short-acting β_2-agonist as required.
● Step 2: low dose inhaled steroids regularly (prevention).
● Step 3: add in long-acting β_2-agonist inhalers (LABA). If no response: stop; if only partial response: increase dose inhaled steroids.
● Step 4: increase inhaled steroid further, or add in either LABA tablet, or slow release theophylline, or leukotriene receptor antagonist (only if upper and lower airway symptoms present).
● Step 5: oral steroid, confirm compliance. Refer to specialist centre where consideration of other forms of immunosuppression may be considered.

Other key points in management.
● Always check inhaler technique.
● Patient should keep PEFR chart.
● Advise regarding lifestyle changes (stop smoking, avoid β blockers, NSAIDs, etc).
● In all patients on long-term oral steroids bone protection should be considered.
● Education, education, education . . .

Management of acute asthma
SEVERE ASTHMA – FEATURES
● Inability to finish sentences.
● RR >25 breaths per minute.
● HR >110 beats per minute.
● PEFR 33–50% expected or patient's best.

LIFE THREATENING ASTHMA – FEATURES
● Silent chest, poor respiratory effort.
● Exhaustion, confusion, coma.
● Bradycardia, hypotension.
● Cyanosis, pO_2 <8 kPa, sats <92%, normal pCO_2.
● PEFR <33% expected or patient's best.

IMMEDIATE MANAGEMENT
● Sit patient up.
● 40–60% oxygen via facemask.
● Nebulisers: 5 mg salbutamol, 0.5 mg ipratropium.
● Oral prednisolone 40–50 mg or hydrocortisone 100 mg every 6 hours.
● If improving, continue oxygen, nebulisers 4–6 hourly, prednisolone PO.

- If not improving, give continuous O_2 + salbutamol nebs, consider IV magnesium sulphate 1.2–2 g over 20 mins or IV aminophylline.
- Refer to ITU – may need intubation.
- On discharge, ensure:
  - patients have an asthma action plan from the nurse specialist
  - PEFR >75% predicted or best with <25% diurnal change
  - sufficient medication for >24 hours
  - good inhaler technique
  - follow-up (GP/asthma nurse two days, respiratory specialist/nurse specialist one month)
  - patient monitor their own PEFR.

3.5. Pneumonia

Can be classified according to *anatomy* (lobar/bronchopneumonia), *source* (community, hospital acquired or aspiration) or *organism*.

MICROBIOLOGICAL CAUSES

- Community-acquired: *Streptococcus pneumoniae, Haemophilus influenzae, Mycoplasma pneumoniae, Chlamydia pneumoniae* and *psittaci, Coxiella burnetii, Legionella pneumophila, Staphylococcus aureus.*
- Hospital-acquired (consider if >48 hours in hospital): Gram negative organisms, *Klebsiella, Pseudomonas, E. coli, Proteus, Staph. aureus*, anaerobes.

CLINICAL FEATURES
Patients with pneumonia are often sick. Symptoms include fever, malaise, lethargy, SOB, cough productive of sputum (rusty = *S. pneumoniae*) and pleuritic chest pain. Ask about pets/birds at home (psittacosis) and hotel visits (*Legionella*). Examination: pyrexia; flushed, warm peripheries (septic); increased respiratory rate and heart rate; decreased oxygen saturations; signs of consolidation (percussion note dull, bronchial breathing, crepitations, pleural rub).

INVESTIGATIONS

- Blood tests: FBC, U&Es (for hyponatraemia secondary to Syndrome of Inappropriate Anti-Diuretic Hormone secretion (SIADH) in 'atypical' pneumonia), LFTs, CRP, clotting; blood film may show red cell agglutination (presence of cold agglutinins = *Mycoplasma*).
- Microbiology: blood cultures, sputum for Gram stain and MC&S, atypical pneumonia blood serology (only if features of atypical pneumonia), urine for pneumococcal and legionella antigen test.
- Other:
  - ABG
  - CXR (for consolidation; consider TB if upper lobes affected)
  - ECG (for AF, SVT due to sepsis).

MANAGEMENT (INCLUDES ABC . . . AS ALWAYS)

- Oxygen therapy, fluid resuscitation, cardiac monitor if unstable.
- Antibiotics: amoxicillin if typical community-acquired or macrolide if 'atypical' organism; give cefuroxime and macrolide IV if severe.
- Chest physiotherapy.
- Tap any suspected effusion/empyema and send for pH (<7.2 suggests empyema), protein concentration, MC&S, AFB and cytology.
- Discuss with ITU/HDU if ≥3 poor prognostic features (**CURB-65**) present:

Confusion (MTS ≤8), **U**rea raised (>7 mmol/l), **R**aised respiratory rate (>30 breaths/min), **B**P systolic <90 mmHg, diastolic <60 mmHg, **A**ge >**65** years.

COMPLICATIONS
- Empyema, lung abscess, pleural effusion, metastatic abscesses, lung fibrosis, death.

Empyema/lung abscess
- **Empyema:** suspect if high spiking temperatures, pleural effusion and no response is seen to antibiotics. Diagnosis is by pleural aspiration. Treatment: chest drain and antibiotics.
- **Lung abscess:** Seen with *S. aureus* and *Klebsiella* pneumonia, aspiration, bronchial obstruction, septic emboli (e.g. IE), spread of subphrenic abscess, pulmonary infarction. Most commonly mixed organisms, frequently *Strep.* species with anaerobes. Treat with broad spectrum antibiotics, surgery is rarely indicated.

3.6. Bronchiectasis
Permanent dilation of the bronchi. Mucus pooling leads to infection usually *S. Aureus* or *H. influenzae*, also *Pseudomonas* (poorer prognosis), with copious sputum production. Clinical features: clubbing; inspiratory and expiratory crackles.

Causes of bronchiectasis
- ○ Congenital: cystic fibrosis (CF), Kartagener's syndrome
- ○ Acquired: following infection (e.g. TB, measles, pertussis), bronchial obstruction, gastric aspiration, allergic broncho-pulmonary aspergillosis, hypogammaglobulinaemia

INVESTIGATIONS
- Sputum MC&S.
- CXR: for cystic areas, fluid levels, thickened bronchial walls; classically 'cysts and tram lines'.
- CT chest: to establish extent of disease, look for signet ring sign.
- Bronchoscopy: if obstruction seen on CT.
- Spirometry: to assess reversibility.
- Establish cause: test for CF, Aspergillus precipitins, cilial function and immunity, consider gastro-oesophageal reflux disease.

TREATMENT
- In acute infection, high dose antibiotics for 14 days.
- If *Pseudomonas* isolated, attempt to eradicate at first isolation.
- Regular postural drainage of mucus.
- Bronchodilators (if reversible airflow obstruction).
- Lobectomy for localised disease.

COMPLICATIONS
- Respiratory: haemoptysis (massive), empyema, abscess, respiratory failure, cor pulmonale, pneumothorax.
- Metastatic abscess formation.
- AA amyloid.

Cystic fibrosis

Common – 1/2500 Caucasian births, carrier rate 1 in 25 (less common in other ethnic groups)

○ **Genetics:** Autosomal recessive, mutation of CF transmembrane conductance regulator gene, chromosome 7 (ΔF508 in 80%). Cells unable to transport chloride leading to secretions with low water and high salt content (mucus is viscous – abnormalities of respiratory tract, pancreas and sweat glands)

○ **Diagnosis:** CF sweat test; genotyping. New-born babies are screened

○ **Complications:** neonates – meconium ileus; children – failure to thrive, pancreatic failure (diabetes, steatorrhoea), recurrent infections/bronchiectasis, biliary disease, infertility

○ **Management:** requires a multidisciplinary team approach. Chest: chest physio, antibiotics. Pancreas: oral pancreatic supplements. Nutritional: advice on diet. Genetic counselling for parents

3.7. Pulmonary embolism (PE)

Occlusion of one or more branches of the pulmonary artery usually by a blood clot from a deep vein thrombosis (DVT). Termed 'massive' if associated with circulatory collapse.

ASSESS CLINICAL PROBABILITY OF PE ON FOLLOWING BASIS:

1. Symptoms (SOB, pleuritic chest pain or haemoptysis) and signs (cyanosis, raised JVP, raised RR, loud P2, pleural rub).
2. Risk factors for PE:
   - major surgery especially abdominal/pelvic surgery
   - obstetrics: pregnancy, post-partum
   - malignancy
   - reduced mobility, e.g. nursing home, hospitalisation
   - previous DVT
   - varicose veins, fracture to lower limb.
3. Alternative explanation can be ruled out, e.g. pneumonia.

RISK ASSESSMENT

- High probability patients: 2 *and* 3 true.
- Intermediate probability patients: 2 *or* 3 true.
- Low probability patients: *neither* 2 *nor* 3 true.

INVESTIGATIONS

- CXR: oligaemic lung fields; wedge-shaped infarct; often normal.
- ECG: sinus tachycardia; AF; right atrial dilatation, right heart strain, RBBB; rarely SI, QIII, TIII.
- ABG: hypoxia, type 1 respiratory failure.
- D-dimers: should *not* be used in patients with high probability of PE. Use in low/intermediate risk depending on local hospital recommendations.
- Computed tomography pulmonary angiography: for non-massive or massive PE.
- Echocardiography is an alternative investigation for massive PE.
- V/Q scan – only if CXR normal and no concurrent pulmonary disease.
- Look for occult malignancy – only if indicated clinically, on CXR or on routine blood tests.
- Consider thrombophilia screen if <50 years with recurrent PE, or strong family history.

MANAGEMENT Initiate treatment if high/intermediate probability <u>before</u> diagnosis is confirmed
- General measures: oxygen therapy, analgesia, cardiac monitor if unwell.
- Anticoagulation:
  - in massive PE: thrombolysis
  - in non-massive PE: low molecular weight (LMW) heparin
  - warfarin once PE is confirmed: three months for temporary risk factors; six months for first idiopathic PE.

PROPHYLAXIS Consider TEDS and prophylactic dose LMW heparin in at-risk patients, e.g. peri-operative patients.

3.8. Pneumothorax

Definition: 'Air within the pleural space'.
- **Primary:** occurring spontaneously in otherwise healthy people; often tall and slim.
- **Secondary:** occurring in patients with underlying lung disease.

CLINICAL FEATURES
- Symptoms: SOB, chest pain (classically worse on inspiration).
- Signs: raised RR, reduced chest expansion, hyper-resonant percussion note, reduced breath sounds on affected side; check trachea is central: if deviated suspect tension pneumothorax (this is a medical emergency).

INVESTIGATIONS CXR to confirm diagnosis (not if tension pneumothorax –a medical emergency).

TREATMENT Primary pneumothorax
- No intervention if not SOB and rim of air <2 cm on CXR.
- If SOB and >2 cm rim of air: attempt simple aspiration.
- If aspiration unsuccessful, proceed to repeat aspiration or intercostal drain.
- If still unsuccessful, refer to respiratory physician within 48 hours or cardiothoracic surgeons after five days for consideration of pleuradhesis.
- On discharge, give advice regarding flying (not for six weeks and risk remains for up to one year) and diving (should be avoided).

Secondary pneumothorax
- If >50 years + >2 cm rim of air on CXR proceed straight to intercostal drain, otherwise attempt aspiration.
- If intercostal drain unsuccessful, then contact respiratory team within 48 hours or cardiothoracic surgeons after three days for consideration of pleuradhesis.
- On discharge, give advise regarding flying and diving (as above).

Tension pneumothorax – *medical emergency*
- ○ Mediastinal shift with tracheal deviation to the contralateral side occurs; cardiorespiratory arrest is imminent
- ○ Patient shows signs of respiratory distress, tachypnoea, tachycardia, shock; tracheal deviation to the contralateral side; reduced breath sounds; hyper-resonance on the affected side
- ○ Initial management: immediate insertion of a large-bore needle into the second intercostal space, in the mid-clavicular line; this buys time for placement of a chest drain (in the 5th intercostal space, anterior mid-axillary line)

3.9. Interstitial lung disease/pulmonary fibrosis
Idiopathic interstitial pneumonias
Cause often unknown: 'idiopathic pulmonary fibrosis' (IPF). Other interstitial pneumonias associated with connective tissue disease (rheumatoid arthritis, SLE, etc.), chronic active hepatitis, ulcerative colitis, lymphoma. IPF has poor prognosis with a mean life expectancy of three years and responds poorly to immunosuppression. The other interstitial pneumonias have variable but better prognosis than IPF.

CLINICAL FEATURES   Patients suffer worsening SOB with respiratory failure, dry cough and weight loss. Signs include clubbing and fine, end-inspiratory crackles.

INVESTIGATIONS
- CXR reveals fibrosis at bases.
- Spirometry: restrictive defect is seen.
- Blood tests: inflammatory markers may be raised, positive autoantibodies in some cases.
- High resolution CT useful for diagnosis.
- Lung biopsy may be indicated.

Occupational lung disease
Asbestos exposure: linked to the shipping industry, builders, factory workers.

CLINICAL PRESENTATION
- Pleural plaques: can develop >20 years post-exposure, a mild restrictive defect only is seen.
- Diffuse pleural thickening: associated with exertional SOB and a restrictive defect.
- Asbestosis: fibrosis in the lower lobes causing dyspnoea; associated risk of developing lung cancer. Compensation is available.
- Lung carcinoma, mesothelioma.

Coal worker's pneumoconiosis: dust particles lodge in small airways, causing small round opacities on CXR, focal emphysema. 'Simple pneumoconiosis' may develop into 'progressive massive fibrosis'.

Occupational asthma: a number of occupational substances have been identified as causing asthma, which may or may not be reversible. Compensation is available.

Hypersensitivity pneumonitis: inhalation of substances, usually spores or avian proteins (farmer's lung, bird fancier's lung), causes a hypersensitivity pneumonitis (type III or IV reaction). Acutely, patients have fever and SOB. Histologically, fibrosis occurs.

Silicosis berylliosis
Other causes of pulmonary fibrosis
- Infections such as TB.
- Sarcoidosis (*see* below).
- Drugs (e.g. amiodarone, methotrexate).
- Radiation.
- Ankylosing spondylitis.
- Allergic bronchopulmonary aspergillosis.

3.10. Sarcoidosis

Cause unknown, multiple systems affected. Incidence: young > old, blacks > whites. Prevalence 30/100,000. Characteristic lesion is the non-caseating granuloma. Presentation: normally insidious onset – asymptomatic, respiratory or systemic symptoms.

DIAGNOSIS   Relies on compatible clinical, radiological and histological findings. Bilateral hilar lymphadenopathy (BHL) and erythema nodosum (EN) in the young is strongly suggestive of sarcoid.

INVESTIGATIONS
- CT may be helpful for diagnosis.
- Transbronchial biopsies useful in select cases.
- Biochemical tests include inflammatory markers, serum ACE (raised in 75% but not diagnostic) and Ca^{2+} (increased vitamin D synthesis). Spirometry reveals a restrictive defect.

Extrapulmonary involvement

- **Skin:** Lupus pernio, EN, nodules
- **Lymphadenopathy**
- **Liver:** biopsy may help clinch diagnosis
- **Splenomegaly**
- **Bone/joints:** arthritis + bone cysts hands/feet
- **Uveitis**
- **Renal:** calculi, nephropathy
- **Cardiac:** cardiomyopathy, effusion or conduction defects
- **Neurological:** cranial nerve palsies, meningitis, space occupying lesion, diabetes insipidus (infiltration of pituitary)
- **Parotid gland enlargement**

MANAGEMENT   Disease progression/regression is monitored via symptoms and serial CXRs, spirometry, serum ACE and Ca^{2+} levels.

Chronic sarcoid may be treated with immunosuppression depending on the organ affected and severity of disease. Pulmonary sarcoid eventually remits in two-thirds, unless extrathoracic disease present.

Acute sarcoidosis or Löfgren's syndrome: fever, arthralgia, EN, BHL on CXR. May resolve with no specific treatment. Prognosis better for acute presentation of sarcoidosis

Differential diagnosis for bilateral hilar lymphadenopathy

- TB
- Lymphoma
- Sarcoid
- Cancer

3.11. Lung cancer
Types (commonest first)
- Squamous cell carcinoma (SCC).
- Small cell lung carcinoma (SCLC): usually metastasised at diagnosis.
- Adenocarcinoma: not linked to smoking, peripheral usually, occurs in sites of fibrosis or scarring ('scar tumour').
- Undifferentiated.

Pancoast's tumour is the name given to an apical tumour causing compression of the C8/T1 nerve roots and pain radiating down the arm. The sympathetic chain is also affected causing Horner's syndrome.

RISK FACTORS
- Unmodifiable: age, male sex.
- Modifiable: smoking, asbestos exposure, pollution (higher rates in urban areas), radiation exposure.

CLINICAL FEATURES
- Respiratory: cough, haemoptysis, SOB, chest pain, wheeze, pleural effusion.
- Systemic: weight loss, lethargy, lymphadenopathy, cachexia.
- Paraneoplastic: e.g. clubbing.
- Horner's syndrome (ptosis, anhydrosis and miosis).

COMPLICATIONS
- Local: pleural effusion, pericarditis, dysphagia (compression from tumour), erosion into rib, phrenic/recurrent laryngeal nerve palsy, Horner's syndrome, superior vena caval (SVC) obstruction, pneumothorax.
- Metastases: to bone, brain, liver, adrenal glands.
- Paraneoplastic: hypertrophic pulmonary osteoarthropathy (HPOA), SIADH, increased ACTH, increased TSH, increased PTH, Eaton-Lambert syndrome.

DIAGNOSIS
- Sputum cytology.
- CXR.
- Staging CT scan.
- Biopsy: transthoracic (CT-guided), bronchoscopy.
- Consider PET scan/bone scan.

STAGING
- SCLC: limited stage disease (i.e. all of the tumour can be treated within a tolerable radiotherapy port); extensive stage disease (metastases in contralateral lung/elsewhere).
- Non-small-cell lung carcinoma (NSCLC): TNM classification.

TREATMENT
- Multidisciplinary approach: involve specialist nurse early.
- SCLC
  - All patients offered multidrug platinum-based chemotherapy.
  - In limited disease: consider radiotherapy as well as chemotherapy +/– prophylactic cranial irradiation if tumour responds to initial treatment.
- NCSLC
  - Stage I and II: offer surgery, if not medically fit offer radical radiotherapy.
  - Stage III and IV: chemotherapy.
  - Stage III can be amenable to surgery or radical radiotherapy.
- Palliation
  - Radiotherapy/chemotherapy may be appropriate to alleviate certain symptoms, e.g. SOB.
  - Dexamethasone for brain metastases.
  - Spinal cord compression: corticosteroids, radiotherapy, surgery where appropriate.

▸ Radiotherapy/chemotherapy/stenting for SVC obstruction.
▸ Symptom control: palliative care input, hospice.

PROGNOSIS Generally poor. SCLC has the worst prognosis, with survival of months

Other types of tumour
- **Carcinoid** – clinical features: wheeze, flushing, diarrhoea. Investigations: 24-hour urine collection for 5-HIAA (5-hydroxy-indolacetic acid) aids diagnosis. Management: curative surgery often possible.
- **Mesotheliomna** – malignancy of the pleura. Poor prognosis.

3.12. Cor pulmonale
Cor pulmonale is right-sided heart failure caused by pulmonary hypertension.

CAUSES
- Chronic hypoxia leading to raised vascular resistance, e.g. COPD, PE.
- High pulmonary blood flow, e.g. left to right shunt.
- Heart disease: e.g. mitral valve disease, HOCM.

DIAGNOSIS
- Based on history of chronic lung disease and history/examination findings of right heart failure.
- CXR shows enlarged right cardiac silhouette and prominent pulmonary artery.
- ECG reveals P-pulmonale, right atrial dilatation, right ventricular strain.

MANAGEMENT
- Treat the underlying condition.
- Long-term oxygen therapy.
- Symptom control: fluid restriction, avoidance of NSAIDs, diuretics.
- Treatment of heart failure (*see* section on *Heart Failure*).
- Surgery: consider heart-lung transplantation.

Primary pulmonary hypertension is a rare condition usually affecting young patients; the patient presents with pulmonary hypertension but no cause is found. Management: refer to a specialist centre for further investigation.

3.13. Respiratory emergencies
See sections on *Asthma*, *COPD*, *PE* and *Pneumothorax*.

Acute respiratory distress syndrome
Can occur secondary to a multitude of severe insults, including severe sepsis and trauma. The resulting pulmonary oedema is non-cardiac. Management: requires treatment of the underlying cause and supportive care (airway management, circulatory support etc).

3.14. Investigations
Arterial blood gases

pH	7.35–7.45 = normal	<7.35 = acidosis
	>7.45 = alkalosis	
serum Bicarbonate (HCO₃)	22–26 = normal	
Base Excess (BE)	+/−2 = normal	
pO_2	>10.6 KPa = normal	Respiratory failure if pO_2 <8 KPa
pCO_2	4.7–6 KPa = normal	

Type 1 respiratory failure: pO_2 <8 KPa and pCO_2 <4.7
Type 2 respiratory failure: pO_2 <8 KPa and pCO_2 >6

Causes of type 1 respiratory failure: any cause of a ventilation-perfusion (V/Q) mismatch, e.g. PE, pneumonia, COPD, asthma.

Causes of type 2 respiratory failure: any cause of type 1 failure plus any cause of hypoventilation such as:
1 neuromuscular conditions – causing weakness of the respiratory muscles, e.g. myasthenia gravis;
2 reduced respiratory drive, e.g. opiates, CNS tumours;
3 thoracic wall defects, e.g. kyphoscoliosis.

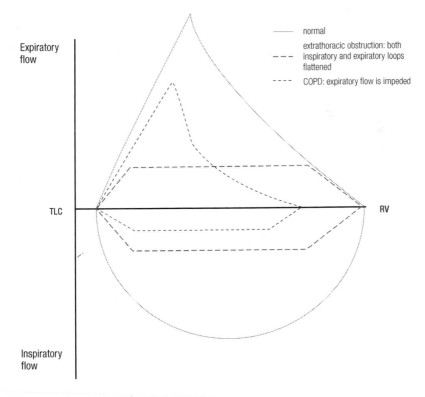

FIGURE 3.1 Flow volume loops.

Peak expiratory flow rate (PEFR) and spirometry

PEFR is a measure of the severity of obstructive airways disease and should be recorded on all patients with asthma and COPD who are admitted with an exacerbation of their condition. Always ensure that the patient's technique is adequate and compare the results to patient's best (if patient knows) or predicted PEFR.

Formal spirometry.

- FEV1 = volume of gas expired in first second of forced expiration (related to PEFR).
- FVC = total volume of gas expired with forced expiration.
- FEV1/FVC <70% = Obstruction.
- FEV1/FVC >70% = Restriction (actual FEV1 and FVC must also be lower than predicted; patients with normal spirometry will have FEV1/FVC >70% also).

Flow-volume loops

Patient inspires rapidly to maximum volume from expiration, then forced expiration is carried out. This produces a flow-volume loop.

Bronchoscopy

Indicated for further investigation of cough, haemoptysis, unusual presentation of chest infection (e.g. if you suspect PCP), for bronchial washings, and to further investigate a lesion resting in the bronchial tree when an endobronchial biopsy is also required. In order to perform, pO_2 needs to be >8k KPa.

CT guided lung biopsy

The procedure of choice if there is a peripheral lesion not amenable to biopsy by bronchoscopy. Risk of pneumothorax $\approx$ 20%, 3% require chest drain.

4

Gastroenterology

4.1. Disorders of the oesophagus
Dysphagia
Difficulty swallowing: classically affects solids more than fluids if obstructive, but early involvement of fluids if neurogenic or a motility problem, e.g. achalasia.

Causes of dysphagia
- ○ **In the lumen:** foreign body
- ○ **In the oesophageal wall:** carcinoma, achalasia, web, stricture, pharyngeal pouch
- ○ **Outside the wall:** mediastinal tumours, retrosternal goitre, left atrial enlargement
- ○ **Neurogenic:** can be broadly classified into cortical causes (e.g. stroke, dementia) and 'peripheral' disorders affecting the anterior horn cell (bulbar palsy in MND, polio), neuromuscular junction (myasthenia gravis) and muscle

Oesophageal carcinoma
Incidence increases with increasing age (peak incidence 50–70 years) and more common in males (3:1). Majority are squamous cell carcinomas ($\approx 85\%$) and the rest are mainly remainder adenocarcinomas which typically arise from the lower $1/3$ from a Barrett's oesophagus.

RISK FACTORS
- Smoking.
- Alcohol.
- Achalasia.
- Barrett's oesophagus (for adenocarcinoma).
- Oesophageal web.

CLINICAL FEATURES (MAY BE ASYMPTOMATIC UNTIL LATE IN DISEASE)
- Progressive dysphagia from solids to liquids.
- Weight loss, loss of appetite.
- Regurgitation +/– cough.
- Few physical signs – cachexia +/– enlarged supraclavicular lymph node.

DIAGNOSIS Made with OGD and biopsy (although can be seen with barium swallow). Further imaging: CT scanning for staging.

MANAGEMENT
- Treatment: surgical resection +/– radiotherapy or chemotherapy.
- Palliative options include endoscopic dilation and stenting.

Overall prognosis is poor ≈ 5% survival rate at five years.

Barrett's oesophagus
Transformation of the lower squamous epithelium of the oesophagus to columnar gastric epithelium. This is a premalignant condition. Predisposing factors: gastro-oesophageal reflux. Presentation: often with dyspepsia or as an incidental finding at endoscopy. Management: regular screening OGD and biopsy for malignant change.

Hiatus hernia
Abnormal protrusion of the the stomach through the oesophageal opening in the diaphragm, leading to a more proximally placed oesophageal-gastric (O-G) junction. ≈ 3/4 are sliding (i.e. the O-G junction and stomach pass through the opening) and 1/4 are rolling (i.e. the O-G junction remains below the opening, with the cardia of the stomach only passing through it). Incidence: very common. Predisposes to gastro-oesophageal reflux. Diagnosis: made on OGD or barium swallow.

Achalasia
An oesophageal disorder characterised by failure of normal peristalsis, failure of relaxation of the lower oesophageal sphincter (LOS) and an increased LOS resting tone; caused by an abnormality of the myenteric plexus.

PRESENTATION Can occur at any age; initial symptom is typically dysphagia (usually to liquids earlier than solids); other symptoms include regurgitation and chest pain.

INVESTIGATIONS Barium swallow shows a dilated tapering oesophagus; oesophageal manometry shows a high LOS resting tone.

MANAGEMENT Conservative unless symptoms are severe. Treatment options include: botox injection; endoscopic LOS dilatation and surgery, e.g. Heller's myotomy.

Gastro-oesophageal reflux disease (GORD)

Caused by failure of the normal anti-reflux mechanisms, e.g. in hiatus hernia. Risk factors: alcohol or caffeine intake, obesity, smoking, pregnancy.

CLINICAL FEATURES
- Retrosternal chest pain ('heartburn') typically worse on lying down.
- Regurgitation of acid/water.

DIAGNOSIS   Made with oesophageal pH monitoring.

MANAGEMENT
- Lifestyle modification: avoid alcohol, stop smoking, weight loss, dietary changes.
- If symptoms persist: H_2 antagonist or PPI and investigate with OGD.
- Surgery (Nissen fundoplication) in select cases.

Oesophageal web (Plummer-Vinson syndrome)

Premalignant condition. More common in women and associated with iron deficiency. Gives rise to symptoms of dysphagia. Management is with iron replacement and endoscopic dilation in select cases.

Oesophageal stricture

Narrowing of the oesophagus, normally presenting with dysphagia. Causes: oesophageal carcinoma, chronic GORD, chemical ingestion. Management: treat underlying cause; consider endoscopic dilatation.

Pharyngeal pouch

Diverticulum of the pharyngeal muscosa through a weakness in the wall between the thryopharyngeus and cricopharyngeus. Presentation: typically with abnormal fetor and dysphagia or complications such as aspiration. Diagnosis is confirmed with barium swallow. Management: pouch can be excised surgically if problematic.

4.2. Disorders of the stomach

Peptic ulcer disease (gastric and duodenal ulcers)

Aetiology: due to acid oversecretion. More common in men (3:1).

RISK FACTORS
- *Helicobacter pylori* infection.
- Smoking.
- Drugs (NSAIDs, corticosteroids).
- Stressful scenarios, e.g. major surgery.

CLINICAL FEATURES
- Dyspepsia, i.e. epigastric pain (classically: gastric ulcers – pain is worse with eating; duodenal ulcers – pain is worse at night/hours after eating).
- Complications: upper GI bleeding (*see* below) and perforation.

INVESTIGATIONS
- In the younger person investigate for *H. pylori* status (e.g. *H.pylori* breath test) with eradication treatment is all that is normally required.
- If >55 years and symptoms are new or persistent +/– associated warning symptoms, e.g. weight loss/anaemia, urgent referral for investigation for

possible gastric carcinoma is necessary (OGD + biopsy + CLO test for *H. pylori* status).

MANAGEMENT
- Remove any precipitating factors.
- Eradicate *H. pylori* if present: triple therapy with a PPI + two antibiotics (e.g. amoxicillin and clarithromycin).
- Consider longer term treatment with PPI.

Gastric carcinoma
More common in males (2:1), aged >50 years old. Usually adenocarcinoma, with the pylorus/antrum being the most commonly affected sites.

RISK FACTORS   Chronic gastric inflammation, *H. pylori* infection, smoking.

CLINICAL FEATURES
- Dyspepsia.
- Weight loss, anorexia.
- Complications: upper GI bleeding or perforation.

INVESTIGATIONS
- OGD + biopsy.
- Staging CT scan.

MANAGEMENT
- Multi-disciplinary approach involving surgeons, oncologists, pain and McMillan teams.
- Surgery (partial or total gastrectomy) – curative if early stage. May also be indicated for palliation in later stages.
- Palliation – if advanced disease.

4.3. Upper gastrointestinal bleed
This refers to haemorrhage arising from the upper gastrointestinal tract proximal to the ligament of Treitz. Usually this is a medical emergency, presenting with haematemesis, coffee-ground vomiting or melaena.

Causes of upper GI bleeding

○ Peptic ulcer disease	○ Gastritis/oesophagitis
○ Oesophageal varices	○ Gastric/oesophageal tumours
○ Mallory-Weiss tear	

PRESENTATION   May be mild, e.g. Mallory-Weiss tear but often bleeding is severe leading to hypovolaemia and shock.

MANAGEMENT
- ABC – high flow oxygen, insert two large bore IV cannulae and fluid resuscitate.
- Send urgent bloods for FBC, U&Es, LFTs, clotting and crossmatch six units blood; transfuse as appropriate.
- Catheterise +/– insert CVP line and monitor closely.
- Give IV PPI +/– vasoactive drug, e.g. vasopressin or octreotide.
- OGD for *diagnosis* of source of bleeding, +/– *intervention*: banding/ sclerotherapy of oesophageal varices; injection of ulcers with adrenaline.

- Consider balloon tamponade (Sengstaken-Blakemore tube) – can provide temporary haemostasis in variceal bleeding.
- Involve ITU and general surgical teams if bleeding is severe/uncontrolled.

4.4. Coeliac disease (gluten-sensitive enteropathy)

Aetiology: gluten intolerance (*Note*: gluten is found in rye, wheat and barley) leading to villous atrophy in the proximal small bowel and consequently malabsorption. Common and often undiagnosed for several years. Associations: increased incidence among those of Irish descent and with certain HLA types, e.g. HLA-B8.

CLINICAL FEATURES
- Diarrhoea/steatorrhoea.
- Weight loss, general malaise.
- Abdominal discomfort +/– nausea/vomiting.
- Anaemia.
- Complications: increased risk of malignancy particularly small bowel lymphoma, dermatitis herpetiformis, peripheral neuropathy.

INVESTIGATIONS AND MANAGEMENT
- Micro- or macrocytic anaemia due to iron or folate deficiency (may have both).
- Autoantibodies: anti-gliadin, anti-endomysial, anti-tissue transglutaminase.
- OGD + jejunal biopsy.
- Management – strict adherence to a gluten-free diet.

4.5. Malabsorption

Usually causes diarrhoea and non-specific symptoms such as weight loss and lethargy.

Causes of malabsorption
- Coeliac disease
- Other causes of villous atrophy, e.g. Whipple's disease
- Small bowel resection
- Bacterial overgrowth
- Chronic GI infections, e.g. giardiasis
- Chronic pancreatitis
- Cystic fibrosis

4.6. Diarrhoea

Multiple definitions: increased amount, increased frequency or decreased consistency of stool.

Causes of diarrhoea
- GI infections – *see ID* section
- Colorectal cancer
- Diverticular disease
- Inflammation, e.g. inflammatory bowel disease
- Malabsorption – *see* above
- Irritable bowel syndrome – *see* below
- Ischaemic colitis
- Drug reactions
- Autonomic neuropathy
- Laxatives

Causes of bloody diarrhoea: inflammatory bowel disease, GI infections (dysentery), colorectal cancer, ischaemic colitis.

4.7. Constipation

Multiple definitions: decreased amount, decreased frequency, or harder stools.

Causes of constipation

○ Obstruction, e.g. colorectal cancer, diverticular disease
○ Decreased motility, e.g. neurological disorders
○ Drugs, e.g. opiates, anticholinergics
○ IBS (a diagnosis of exclusion)
○ Low-fibre diet

Investigation and treatment of the underlying cause is necessary; laxatives can be useful for symptomatic relief. Types of laxatives include: bulk-forming agents, faecal softeners, stimulants (e.g. senna), or osmotics (e.g. lactulose).

4.8. Inflammatory bowel disease (IBD)

Peak incidence is between the ages of 20 to 40 years. Two disorders cause chronic inflammation and although there is overlap they have distinct features:
- **Crohn's disease.**
- **Ulcerative Colitis (UC).**

Both conditions are associated with HLA-B27 and ankylosing spondylitis. In addition, there is an increased risk of colorectal cancer (more for UC than Crohn's).

Crohn's disease

Incidence M=F. Can affect any area of the GI tract from the mouth to the anus. The terminal ileum is the most commonly affected site. Different areas of bowel can be affected at the same time with normal bowel intervening, i.e. skip lesions.

HISTOLOGICALLY Transmural disease (i.e. whole thickness of the bowel is affected) with non-caeseating granuloma.

CLINICAL FEATURES
- Abdominal pain (often right iliac fossa).
- Weight loss.
- Diarrhoea (may be bloody).
- Fever, malaise and anorexia in acute episodes ('flare-ups').
- Aphthous ulcers (mouth/anus).
- Perianal skin tags, abscesses and fistulae.
- Malabsorption (e.g. of vitamin B12 due to terminal ileal disease).
- Anaemia (which can be due to iron or B12 deficiency).
- Extra-intestinal disease:
  - clubbing
  - arthritis
  - nephrolithiasis
  - eye problems (e.g. uveitis)
  - skin disorders (e.g. erythema nodosum).

INVESTIGATIONS
- Barium follow-through (to image small intestine) or barium enema (to

image large intestine) – for strictures or ulceration (so-called 'cobblestone' appearance).
- Upper GI endoscopy/colonoscopy (depending on symptoms) +/– biopsy.

Ulcerative colitis (UC)
Involves the large bowel only (although the terminal ileum can also be affected in a 'backwash ileitis'). The rectum is always involved and the disease progresses proximally.

HISTOLOGICALLY Only the mucosa and submucosa are involved with ulceration and the presence of crypt abscesses, pseudopolyps and goblet cell depletion.

CLINICAL FEATURES
- Bloody diarrhoea with mucus.
- Abdominal pain.
- Weight loss.
- Anaemia (usually due to iron deficiency).
- Extra-intestinal disease: skin disorders (e.g. pyoderma gangrenosum), increased incidence of primary sclerosing cholangitis.
- Complications: toxic megacolon in acute presentations +/– perforation.

INVESTIGATIONS
- Sigmoidoscopy or colonoscopy + biopsy.
- Barium enema: shows loss of haustra ('lead pipe' colon), pseudopolyps.
- If suspect toxic megacolon then serial abdominal x-rays should be performed to monitor progression/resolution.

MANAGEMENT: SIMILAR FOR BOTH CROHN'S DISEASE AND UC
- Hospital admission may be required for acute 'flare-ups': fluid resuscitation and steroids +/– antibiotics +/– serial AXR if toxic megacolon; and surgery may form part of the management.
- Medical treatment options:
  - aminosalicylates, e.g. mesalazine and olsalazine
  - steroids, e.g. oral prednisolone or topical for proctitis
  - steroid-sparing agents, e.g. azathioprine
  - newer agents, e.g. infliximab (anti-TNF-alpha).
- Surgery: indicated if recurrent obstructive symptoms and fistulae.

Irritable bowel syndrome (IBS)
Functional bowel disorder. Diagnosis of exclusion. More common in women.

CLINICAL FEATURES
- Abdominal pain +/– bloating typically relieved by defaecation or the passage of wind.
- Alternating bouts of constipation and diarrhoea.

MANAGEMENT
- Exclude other bowel pathology then reassure.
- Advise dietary modifications, e.g. high fibre diet and antispasmodics, e.g. mebeverine.

4.9. Jaundice

Yellow pigmentation of the skin, sclera and mucous membranes due to an accumulation of unconjugated or conjugated bilirubin. Observed clinically when the serum bilirubin is >30 µmol/l. Can be classified as pre-hepatic, hepatic or post-hepatic (cholestatic or obstructive)

Pre-hepatic jaundice

Occurs due to excess bilirubin production from any cause. Plasma bilirubin is predominantly unconjugated.

Causes of pre-hepatic jaundice

○ Haemolysis, e.g. haemolytic anaemia (*see* Haematology section for causes)
○ Neonatal jaundice

Hepatic jaundice

Occurs due to hepatocellular damage. Normally both unconjugated and conjugated bilirubin are present in the plasma.

Causes of hepatic jaundice

○ Viral hepatitis (hepatitis A, B, C, D and E, CMV, EBV)
○ Alcohol
○ Liver metastases
○ Cirrhosis (*see* below)
○ Drugs, e.g. paracetamol
○ Metabolic, e.g. Wilson's disease, haemochromatosis, alpha-1-antitrypsin deficiency
○ Autoimmune, e.g. autoimmune hepatitis

Post-hepatic jaundice

Due to obstruction of the bile ducts either intra- or extrahepatically (cholestasis) (*see Obstructive jaundice* section under *General Surgery*). Primarily conjugated bilirubin found in the plasma.

Note there are a number of congenital disorders that cause jaundice: Gilbert's syndrome (relatively common and otherwise asymptomatic, jaundice may only appear during intercurrent illness), Crigler-Najjar syndrome, Dubin-Johnson syndrome, Rotor's syndrome.

CLINICAL FEATURES
- Yellow pigmentation of the sclera, skin and mucous membranes.
- Take a detailed history for: recent blood transfusion, body piercing, intravenous drug abuse, jaundiced contacts, sexual history, recent travel abroad, excess alcohol intake, drug use (including non-prescription).
- Look for signs of underlying disease causing jaundice, e.g. chronic liver disease.

INVESTIGATIONS   Initial investigations.
- LFTs: raised bilirubin (check if unconjugated or conjugated). If ALT and AST high, then likely hepatic jaundice; if ALP and GGT raised, then likely obstructive jaundice.
- Urinalysis: pre-hepatic – increased urobilinogen but no bilirubin; obstructive – no urobilinogen but positive for bilirubin.
- Abdominal ultrasound for cholelithiasis, hepatomegally etc.

Further investigations are guided by findings on initial investigation.

- Pre-hepatic: investigate for haemolysis: *see Haematology* section.
- Hepatic: 'Liver screen': viral serology (A, B, C, CMV, EBV), serum ferritin/iron studies (for haemochromatosis), copper/caeruloplasmin (for Wilson's disease), autoantibodies (ANA, anti-mitochondrial, anti-smooth muscle), AFP (raised in hepatocellular carcinoma); consider liver biopsy.
- Post-hepatic: depends on ultrasound findings: if evidence of duct dilation, patient will need MRCP +/− ERCP; Consider CT abdomen if no gallstones seen and cancer of the pancreas suspected; if no duct dilation consider liver biopsy.

4.10. Ascites

Accumulation of free fluid within the peritoneal cavity. Can be classified as either a transudate (<30 g/l) or an exudate (>30 g/l) depending on protein content.

Causes of ascites

- ○ **Exudate** (*mnemonic is IMP*): Infection (bacterial or TB), Malignancy, Pancreatitis
- ○ **Transudate** (*mnemonic is PRINT*): Portal hypertension (e.g. due to cirrhosis), Right-sided heart failure, IVC obstruction, Nephrotic syndrome, Thrombosis of the portal vein (Budd-Chiari syndrome)

On examination: there is abdominal distension with evidence of shifting dullness.

INVESTIGATIONS Investigate for underlying cause: perform diagnostic ascitic tap (for albumin, total protein, amylase, blood, WCC, MC&S and cytology).

MANAGEMENT Treat underlying cause. Consider paracentesis (+/− IV albumin replacement) for tense ascites. For transudates: fluid restriction, low salt intake and diuretics, e.g. spironolactone, may be helpful.

4.11. Cirrhosis

This is irreversible liver damage, characterised and defined histologically by loss of normal liver architecture, fibrosis and nodular regeneration and represents the final pathway for a number of chronic liver diseases.

Causes of cirrhosis

- ○ Alcohol
- ○ Hepatitis B, B and D, or C
- ○ Autoimmune hepatitis
- ○ Cryptogenic (idiopathic)
- ○ Metabolic: haemochromatosis, Wilson's disease, alpha-1 anti-trypsin deficiency
- ○ Primary biliary cirrhosis

CLINICAL FEATURES There may be signs of chronic liver disease (although some patients will have no signs).

- Jaundice.
- Hands: clubbing, leuconychia, Dupuytren's contracture, palmar erythema.
- Asterixis ('liver flap').
- Foetor hepaticus.
- Over upper body: spider naevi (>5 is abnormal), gynaecomastia, loss of axillary hair, caput medusae (distended abdominal veins).
- On abdominal and genital exam: ascites, liver is usually small and not palpable, testicular atrophy, loss of pubic hair.

COMPLICATIONS   Portal hypertension (*see* below), hepatic encephalopathy, hepatorenal syndrome, hepatocellular carcinoma, ascites.

Portal hypertension

Commonly due to cirrhosis but other causes include portal vein thrombosis, Budd-Chiari syndrome and heart disease (right-sided heart failure, constrictive pericarditis). May be asymptomatic or present with:
- varices with a risk of subsequent upper GI bleeding
- ascites
- splenomegaly

INVESTIGATIONS
- Blood tests: abnormal LFTs, hypoalbuminaemia, abnormal clotting.
- Tests to identify the cause.
- Abdominal ultrasound.
- Liver biopsy – required for definitive diagnosis.

MANAGEMENT
- Treat the underlying cause (e.g. alcohol cessation) and complications.
- Refer to a specialist for consideration for liver transplantation in select cases.

4.12. Chronic hepatitis

Inflammation of the liver lasting longer than six months. Often classified into two types:

Chronic persistent hepatitis

Relatively benign and patients normally recover spontaneously over months to years. Patients are generally asymptomatic without signs of chronic liver disease. Blood tests: show raised ALT and AST. Cause in the majority of cases is viral hepatitis (B, B+D or C).

Chronic active hepatitis

Normally progresses to cirrhosis and liver failure. Histologically, piecemeal and bridging necrosis of the liver with later fibrosis seen. Blood tests: show raised ALT and AST. Causes include: alcohol, hepatitis B, B+D or C, autoimmune hepatitis, haemochromatosis, Wilson's disease, alpha-1 anti-trypsin deficiency.

4.13. Alcoholic liver disease (ALD)

Alcohol may cause a number of problems of increasing severity in the liver:
- Alcoholic steatosis – fatty change, reversible if patient stops drinking.
- Alcoholic hepatitis – may present acutely with jaundice, tender hepatomegaly, vomiting, fever and general malaise.
- Alcoholic cirrhosis.

INVESTIGATIONS
- Abnormal LFTs: raised bilirubin, AST >ALT, GGT; raised serum ferritin.
- Liver biopsy.

MANAGEMENT
- Abstinence from alcohol (and if acute presentation, treatment of withdrawal).
- Treatment of complications of cirrhosis.
- Surgery: consider liver transplantation in select cases.

4.14. Autoimmune hepatitis

More common in women (3:1), and presents from a young age. Associated with other autoimmune conditions, e.g. Hashimoto's thyroiditis, Sjögren's syndrome and ulcerative colitis. Presentation: produces a chronic active hepatitis with insidious onset of features of chronic liver disease. A minority of patients present with an acute hepatitis.

INVESTIGATIONS
- Signs of inflammation: raised ESR/CRP.
- Abnormal LFTs: raised bilirubin, AST and ALT (and later on low albumin).
- Raised serum IgG.
- ANA and anti-smooth muscle antibodies present in the majority of cases, anti-liver and kidney microsomal (LKM) antibodies may also be present.
- Liver biopsy may show signs of chronic active hepatitis.

MANAGEMENT
- Medical therapy: prednisolone +/– azathioprine.
- Treat complications of cirrhosis.
- Surgical: consider liver transplantation.

4.15. Metabolic liver disease

Wilson's disease

Rare, inherited autosomal recessive disorder of copper metabolism (ATP 7B on chromosome 13), leading to the accumulation of copper, e.g. liver, basal ganglia.

CLINICAL FEATURES
- Liver disease: acute or chronic active hepatitis, cirrhosis.
- Neurological disease: extrapyramidal syndrome most common presentation.
- Eyes: Kayser-Fleischer rings (deposition of copper in Descemet's membrane).

INVESTIGATIONS AND MANAGEMENT
- Abnormal LFTs.
- Reduced serum caeruloplasmin (and usually reduced serum copper).
- 24 hour urine collection: excess urinary copper excretion.
- Liver biopsy demonstrates copper deposition.
- Medical therapy: penicillamine is first line.
- Treat complications of cirrhosis.
- Surgery: consider liver transplantation.

Haemochromatosis

An inherited autosomal recessive disorder of iron uptake (HFE on chromosome 6), leading to excess iron deposition.

CLINICAL FEATURES
- Liver disease.
- Skin: bronze pigmentation.
- Pancreas: diabetes.
- Heart: cardiomyopathy.
- Joints: arthritis.

INVESTIGATIONS AND MANAGEMENT
- Abnormal LFTs; raised serum ferritin and iron.

- Liver biopsy demonstrates iron deposition.
- Venesection to reduce iron load.
- Screening close family members.
- Treat complications of cirrhosis.
- Surgery: consider liver transplantation.

Alpha-1 anti-trypsin deficiency
Autosomal recessive disorder (chromosome 14).

CLINICAL FEATURES
- Liver disease.
- Lung disease: emphysema.

INVESTIGATIONS AND MANAGEMENT
- Blood tests: abnormal LFTs; low serum alpha-1 anti-trypsin.
- Lung function tests.
- Imaging: CT chest shows emphysema.
- Liver biopsy.
- Treat complications of cirrhosis and consider liver transplantation.

4.16. Other liver disease
Primary biliary cirrhosis
Autoimmune disease – may be associated with other autoimmune diseases. Majority of cases affect females, with onset at >40 years. Presentation: insidious onset – often asymptomatic at diagnosis or non-specific symptoms of fatigue.

CLINICAL FEATURES
- Obstructive (cholestatic) jaundice with pruritus.
- Xanthelasma, hepatomegaly, splenomegaly, skin pigmentation.
- May progress to cirrhosis and features of chronic liver disease.

INVESTIGATIONS AND MANAGEMENT
- Abnormal LFTs: raised ALP +/– mildly raised bilirubin, AST/ALT.
- Raised serum IgM; serum anti-mitochondrial antibodies present in 95%.
- Liver biopsy.
- Medical Therapy:
  - treat symptoms, e.g. colestyramine for pruritis
  - ursodeoxycholic acid.
- Treat complications of cirrhosis and consider liver transplantation.

Primary sclerosing cholangitis
Rare. More common in men. Clinical features: fatigue, pruritus, jaundice, abdominal pain and/or pyrexia. On examination: hepatomegaly and/or splenomegaly +/– features of chronic liver disease. Patients with ulcerative colitis are at increased risk. Investigations: raised ALP, AST, ALT and bilirubin, hypergammaglobulinaemia and positive p-ANCA autoantibodies. ERCP reveals multiple strictures within the biliary tree (giving a beaded appearance). Liver biopsy should be performed. Management: treat symptoms, e.g. pruritis with colestyramine, ursodeoxycholic acid. Consider liver transplantation in end stage disease.

Hepatocellular carcinoma (HCC)
In most cases there is pre-existing cirrhosis and HCC should be considered in

all patients with cirrhosis that suddenly deteriorates. More common in males. Investigations: raised serum alpha-foetoprotein (AFP); abdominal ultrasound or CT +/– biopsy will aid diagnosis. If detected early consider hepatic resection. Transplantation is an option, but for many patients treatment is palliative, e.g. chemotherapy, ethanol injection.

4.17. Hepatosplenomegaly

Causes of hepatosplenomegally

- ○ **Hepatomegaly** (*mnemonic CHA*): carcinoma (secondary), cardiac failure (right), cirrhosis (early on although generally small as disease progresses), hepatitis (e.g. alcohol), haematological disease (e.g. CML), alcoholic liver disease
- ○ **Splenomegaly:** CML, myelofibrosis, kala-azar, malaria (all cause massive), right cardiac failure, portal hypertension, storage diseases, haemolytic anaemia
- ○ **Hepatosplenomegaly:** haematological disease (e.g. lymphoproliferative and myelo-proliferative disorders), portal hypertension with chronic liver disease, infections (e.g. viral hepatitis), amyloid

4.18. Acute liver failure

Acute, severe impairment of liver function within six months of onset of symptoms of liver disease, with hepatic encephalopathy and/or coagulopathy. Can be classified as **fulminant**, i.e. within 8 weeks from the initial onset of symptoms, or **subfulminant**, if the interval is >8 weeks but <6 months.

Causes of acute liver failure

- ○ **Drug-related:** paracetamol overdose or other drug reactions
- ○ **Viral hepatitis:** mainly hepatitis B
- ○ **Vascular:** e.g. Budd-Chiari syndrome, hypoperfusion in shock
- ○ **Other:** malignant infiltration, autoimmune liver disease, Wilson's disease

CLINICAL FEATURES   Jaundice, hepatic encephalopathy, coagulopathy, renal failure (hepatorenal syndrome), sepsis, hypoglycaemia, hypoxia.

Hepatic encephalopathy (grades 1–4)

- ○ **Grade 1:** Altered mood/behaviour
- ○ **Grade II:** Increased drowsiness, confusion, slurred speech
- ○ **Grade III:** Stupor, incoherence, restlessness, significant confusion
- ○ **Grade IV:** Coma

INVESTIGATIONS
- FBC (for thrombocytopenia), U&Es (for hepatorenal syndrome).
- LFTs – ALT/AST significantly raised; bilirubin – useful prognostic indicator.
- Glucose (often low).
- Clotting (INR >1.5).
- Blood cultures.
- Investigate for underlying cause, e.g. paracetamol levels, viral serology.
- Arterial blood gas (for hypoxia and acidosis).
- Abdominal ultrasound.

MANAGEMENT

- ABC and consider transfer to ITU. Insert urinary catheter, CVP line and NG tube and monitor closely.
- Avoid drugs metabolised by the liver and sedatives.
- Treat underlying cause, e.g. N-acetyl cysteine in paracetamol toxicity – this may also have a role in other forms of liver disease.
- Treat complications, e.g. bleeding (correct clotting and transfuse appropriately), hypoglycaemia, seizures, sepsis and malnutrition.
- Assess prognostic factors: degree of encephalopathy, prothrombin time, age and cause of acute liver failure.
- Refer to a specialist liver unit and consider liver transplantation.

5

Renal disease

5.1. Acute renal failure

Rise in creatinine or fall in glomerular filtration rate occurring over hours or days.

Causes of acute renal failure

Pre-renal
- ○ **Hypovolaemia:** e.g. dehydration, bleeding
- ○ **Renal hypoperfusion:** e.g. renal artery stenosis, non-steroidal anti-inflammatory drugs, ACE-inhibitors, angiotensin receptor blockers (ARBs)
- ○ **Hypotension:** e.g. shock
- ○ **Oedematous states:** e.g. CCF, nephritic syndrome

Renal
- ○ **Glomerular disease:** e.g. ANCA-positive glomerulonephritis, lupus, anti-GBM disease
- ○ **Interstitial nephritis:** drugs, infiltrative (lymphoma), granulomatous (sarcoid, TB), infection
- ○ **Tubular injury:** ATN; toxins, e.g. contrast, raised creatine kinase causing rhabdomyolysis; metabolic, e.g. light chains; crystals
- ○ **Vascular:** vasculitis, polyarteritis nodosa, cryoglobulinaemia, cholesterol emboli, renal artery/vein thrombosis

Post-renal – *obstruction to urine flow downsteam of the kidneys*
- ○ In the tube: e.g. ureteric stone
- ○ In the tube wall: e.g. ureteric tumour, bladder tumour obstructing ureteric orifices
- ○ Outside the tube: e.g. prostatic hypertrophy, retroperitoneal fibrosis

CLINICAL FEATURES
- Uraemia: nausea/vomiting, reduced appetite, weight loss, pruritis (itching), fatigue, confusion. Uraemic tinge to skin, raised respiratory rate (metabolic acidosis with respiratory compensation), pericardial rub.
- Pulmonary oedema/fluid overload or hypovolaemia/fluid depletion.

Specific symptoms/signs of the disease process

○ Look for sepsis, hypovolaemia, GI bleed (pre-renal)
○ History of UTIs (reflux)/hypertension/diabetes (likely to point to a more chronic process)
○ Ask about lower urinary tract symptoms, history of renal stones
○ Joint pains/rash/scleritis/serositis (lupus or vasculitis)
○ Back pain (myeloma)
○ Haemoptysis (anti-GBM disease or ANCA-positive vasculitis)
○ URTI (post-infectious GN)
○ Haematuria (IgA nephropathy)
○ PR bleeding/abdominal pain (Henoch-Schönlein Purpura)
○ Recent contrast load (contrast nephropathy)
○ Drug use: e.g. NSAIDs, penicillin
○ Family history: e.g. adult polycystic kidney disease (points to chronicity)
○ Country of origin: e.g. Africa – ?HIV, sickle cell disease or malaria

INVESTIGATIONS   Always attempt to obtain previous renal function from GP or old records – it may reveal that presentation is, in fact, of chronic renal failure. Perform full 'renal screen' to identify the cause of the renal disease.

'Renal screen'

○ Blood tests: ANA, ANCA, anti-GBM, dsDNA, rheumatoid factor, anti-streptolysin titres, complement levels, serum paraprotein, CK (rhabdomyolysis), hepatitis B/C titres, consider HIV, blood cultures, blood film, and haemolysis screen if suspect haemolytic uraemic syndrome (HUS)/thrombotic thrombocytopenic purpura (TTP)
○ Urine: dip for blood and protein, microscopy (casts, WCC, RBC, pus) and culture, Bence-Jones protein (urinary free light chains in myeloma), protein/creatinine ratio for urinary protein quantification
○ Ultrasound: to rule out obstruction and for kidney size (if small ?chronic)
○ CT renal angiography/MRA if renal artery stenosis suspected
○ Consider renal biopsy

ASSESSMENT OF PATIENT IN THE ACUTE SETTING

● ABG: for metabolic acidosis, oxygenation (if pulmonary oedema), quick test for serum potassium level.
● Urgent bloods for: particularly U&Es, LFTs, albumin (low in nephrotic syndrome), clotting, FBC (for Hb and platelet count) and blood film (HUS/TTP).
● Perform full renal screen (as above).
● CXR: for pericardial effusion, pulmonary oedema or haemorrhage.
● ECG: for changes related to hyperkalaemia/HT (clue to diagnosis).

MANAGEMENT

● Fluid resuscitate if dehydrated, aim for euvolaemia.
● Insert CVP line if appropriate – aim for a CVP between 10–12.
● Insert urinary catheter.
● Treat hyperkalaemia – with dextrose/insulin infusion and 10 ml 10% calcium gluconate (cardiac monitor required).
● Treat pulmonary oedema.
● Treat metabolic acidosis (consider sodium bicarbonate IV or PO).
● Consider acute haemodialysis. Indications include:
  ▸ hyperkalaemia

- severe metabolic acidosis
- pulmonary oedema not responding to medical treatment
- uraemic symptoms.
- Treat the cause, liaise with the renal physicians early.
  - With pre-renal causes, support the circulation, i.e. rehydrate, give blood as required, treat sepsis, consider inotropes.
  - With renal failure: target the cause (e.g. immunosuppression for vasculitis).
  - With post-renal: relieve the obstruction.

5.2. Chronic renal failure

Causes of chronic renal failure (CRF)

- ○ Hypertension (HT)
- ○ Diabetes mellitus (DM)
- ○ Glomerulonephritis (GN)*
- ○ Hereditary conditions: e.g. adult polycystic kidney disease
- ○ Renovascular disease (RVD)
- ○ Reflux nephropathy
- ○ Chronic interstitial nephritis
- ○ Drugs: e.g. ciclosporin, lithium, NSAIDs
- ○ Obstructive uropathy
- ○ Amyloidosis
- ○ Sarcoidosis
- ○ Urological causes: e.g. neurogenic bladder
- ○ Posterior urethral valves
- ○ Any cause of ARF may lead to CRF

Glomerulonephritides*

- ○ IgA nephropathy
- ○ Membranous nephropathy
- ○ Minimal change disease
- ○ Focal segmental glomerulosclerosis
- ○ Post-infectious GN
- ○ Membranoproliferative/mesangiocapillary GN
- ○ Rapidly progressive, Crescentic (includes ANCA-positive vasculitis, lupus, can *see* with IgA nephropathy)

STAGES OF CHRONIC KIDNEY DISEASE (CKD)

Stage 1: GFR >90 ml/min but other evidence of disease, e.g. proteinuria
Stage 2: GFR 60–90 ml/min
Stage 3: GFR 30–60 ml/min
Stage 4: GFR 15–30 ml/min
Stage 5: GFR <15 ml/min

HISTORY AND EXAMINATION

- If diabetic, ask about complications such as retinopathy or neuropathy – if present then likely diabetic nephropathy also; if not present then search for another cause of CKD.
- Ask about MIs, CVAs, intermittent claudication, listen for carotid/renal/femoral bruits (atheroma in other vessels suggests atheroma in the renal arteries).
- Is there a history of UTIs (reflux), renal stones, lower urinary tract symptoms?
- Is there a history of Haematuria (IgA nephropathy)?

- Are there symptoms/signs of vasculitis: rash, scleritis, joint pains, etc; URTI (post-infectious)?
- Is there a family history (APKD – palpable kidneys, Alport's syndrome)?
- Take a drug history (NSAIDs, lithium)?
- Is there a history of smoking; travel (HIV)?
- Finally, look for evidence of uraemia and fluid overload.

INVESTIGATIONS
- Blood tests: renal screen; anaemia screen (anaemia is due to lack of erythropoietin production by the kidney); serum bicarbonate, Ca^{2+}, phosphate and PTH (as active form of vitamin D is not produced by the failing kidneys, affecting bone metabolism); glucose/HbA1c.
- Urine: urinalysis – for blood (may indicate IgA nephropathy, active inflammation or simply HT/DM); MC&S; protein : creatinine ratio for proteinuria.
- ECG (for hypertensive changes).
- Imaging:
  - ultrasound to rule out obstruction and assess kidney size
  - CT renal angiography, MRA for renal artery stenosis
  - CXR (for pulmonary oedema).

MANAGEMENT
Treatment of disease process.
- Hypertensive nephropathy – treat aggressively with antihypertensives.
- RVD – consider angioplasty and stenting.
- Diabetic nephropathy – tight control diabetes; reduce proteinuria with ACE-inhibitor +/– ARBs, e.g. candesartan.
    Note: significant proteinuria due to any disease process will speed the progression of CRF, so needs to be reduced.
- Optimise cardiovascular risk factors: excellent BP, diabetic, and cholesterol control and abstinence from smoking will slow the progression to stage 5 CKD.
- Salt restriction and fluid restriction: if fluid overloaded – will help hypertension also.
- Bone health: control phosphate with low phosphate diet and phosphate binders (aim for serum level <1.8 mmol/L), replace vitamin D according to PTH and Ca^{2+} levels.
- Hyperkalaemia: refer to dietitian for low potassium diet.
- Anaemia: aim Hb 11–13 g/dl with IV iron if iron-deplete and recombinant SC erythropoietin therapy.
- Metabolic acidosis: treat with oral sodium bicarbonate to keep serum bicarbonate >20 mmol/L (also helps with treating hyperkalaemia).
- Education for renal replacement therapy (RRT): if renal function poor (GFR <20 ml/min) or deteriorating rapidly, prepare for RRT (options are peritoneal dialysis, haemodialysis or transplantation).

Complications of CRF
○ Progression to stage 5 CKD, end-stage renal failure
○ Increased cardiovascular risk (CRF is an independent risk factor)
○ Fluid overload
○ Hyperkalaemia
○ Anaemia
○ Renal osteodystrophy

○ Secondary and tertiary hyperparathyroidism
○ Metabolic acidosis

5.3. Nephrotic syndrome

Defined as:
- Proteinuria >3 g/day.
- Hypoalbuminaemia.
- Oedema.
- Hypercholesterolaemia.

Causes of nephrotic syndrome (think 'M')

○ Diabetes Mellitus
○ Membranous GN (primary or secondary to other disease processes)
○ Minimal change disease
○ Mesangiocapillary GN
○ AMyloid (AL or AA)
○ Myeloma
○ Also: HIV, focal segmental glomerulosclerosis, IgA nephropathy, SLE Class V

HISTORY AND EXAMINATION   Should be aimed at diagnosing the cause, e.g. back pain may suggest myeloma; there may be a history of DM or of SLE. Haematuria may suggest IgA nephropathy.

INVESTIGATIONS
- Urinalysis (proteinuria).
- Estimation of urinary protein leak* (protein creatinine ratio/24 hour collection).
- Full renal screen and fasting serum cholesterol.
- Ultrasound of the renal tract.
- Renal biopsy.

*Estimation of urinary protein leak was traditionally done with a 24 hour urinary protein collection which is inaccurate. Many renal units now send urine for protein creatinine ratio or PCR: this will give you an estimation of the 24 hour protein leak but from a single urine sample.

MANAGEMENT
- Treat the underlying cause: e.g. steroids in minimal change disease; good diabetic control in DM.
- Treat the oedema: fluid restrict, low salt diet, diuretics. Monitor progress with input/output charts and daily weights. Aim to lose one litre (1 kg) per day.
- Reduce proteinuria with ACE-inhibitor +/– ARB (slows progression of renal disease).
- Reduce cardiovascular risk with BP and cholesterol control, DM control, smoking cessation advice. Statin therapy is usually required due to a very elevated cholesterol.
- If albumin <20 g/L, patient is at risk of DVT/PE or renal vein thrombosis, therefore formally anticoagulate (reason: antithrombin III and other factors are lost along with other proteins via the glomerulus). Suspect renal vein thrombosis if RF deteriorates, back pain, and blood on urine dip – arrange renal vein Doppler ultrasound.

5.4. Renal tubular disease

Tubular defects lead to loss of electrolytes and other substances usually reabsorbed by the tubules.

Renal tubular acidosis (RTA)

Type 1 – Distal
○ Relatively common; seen in a host of renal diseases, genetic and acquired
○ Unable to acidify urine, urine pH >5.3
○ Serum bicarbonate low
○ Complicated by nephrocalcinosis, calculi

Type 2 – Proximal
○ Rare – may be idiopathic or secondary to other renal disease
○ Failure of bicarbonate reabsorption
○ Urine pH, serum bicarbonate variable
○ Complicated by osteomalacia/rickets

RTA type 4 is commonly associated with DM and causes hyperkalaemia and metabolic acidosis (urine pH usually <5.3), secondary to hyporeninaemic hypoaldosteronism.

Fanconi syndrome

Associated with multiple proximal tubular defects leading to glycosuria, aminoaciduria, phosphaturia and RTA. Multiple myeloma should be excluded.

Nephrogenic diabetes insipidus (see *Endocrine* section)

Bartter's syndrome

Severe hypokalaemia secondary to defect in chloride reabsorption leading to salt wasting, particularly seen in children.

Liddle's syndrome

Autosomal dominant. Clinical features: HT and hypokalaemia.

Gitelman's syndrome

Autosomal recessive. Clinical features: hypokalaemia, hypomagnesaemia and hypocalciuria.

Nephrocalcinosis

Deposition of calcium usually in the renal medulla. Causes: hypercalcaemia associated with hypercalciuria (e.g. hyperparathyroidism, sarcoid), idiopathic hypercalciuria, distal RTA, oxalosis, medullary sponge kidney.

5.5. Inherited renal diseases
Adult polycystic kidney disease (APKD)

● Autosomal dominant (chromosomes 16 (PKD 1) and 4 (PKD 2)); due to an abnormality of polycystin 1 and polycystin 2.
● Incidence: affects 1 in 1000.
● Clinical features: cysts in kidneys, liver, pancreas.
● Complications: abdominal pain, bleeding/infection in cyst, calculi, UTIs, end-stage renal disease, cerebral aneurysms, HT.
● Diagnosis: ultrasound; gene linkage analysis (not usually necessary).

- Further investigations: if there is family history of brain haemorrhage or patient suffers headaches then exclude berry aneurysms with imaging, e.g. MRA brain.

Autosomal recessive polycystic kidney disease
- Rare, presents in childhood, associated with chromosome 6.

Tuberous sclerosis
- Autosomal dominant (chromosomes 9 and 16).
- Clinical features.
  - Angiomyolipomas in kidneys (can cause retroperitoneal haemorrhage), cortical tubers (brain), retinal hamartomas, cardiac rhabdomyomas.
  - Skin: adenoma sebaceum (facial angiofibromas), ash leaf spots (hypopigmented macules), shagreen patches (lumbosacral area) and periungal fibromas.

Von Hippel-Lindau disease
- Autosomal dominant (chromosome 3).
- Clinical features: retinal angiomas, cerebellar and spinal haemangioblastomas, phaeochromocytomas, and renal cell carcinomas.
- Management: screen yearly with ophthalmoscopy. Other screening investigations include MRI brain/spine/abdomen and contrast CT abdomen.

Alport's syndrome
- Usually X-linked, but may be autosomal recessive or autosomal dominant.
- Patients have an abnormal glomerular basement membrane due to an abnormality in type IV collagen, against which anti-GBM antibodies are directed.
- Clinical features: deafness, eye involvement, microscopic haematuria, nephritic syndrome, CRF.

5.6. Acid-base balance
Metabolic acidosis
On ABG: pH <7.35, BE < –2, HCO_3^- < 22 mmol/L

Anion gap = (serum Na^+ + K^+) – (serum Cl^- + HCO_3^-).

Calculate the anion gap. If increased then there is an excess of unmeasured anions/acid in the blood.

Treatment: depends on the cause.

Causes of *increased* anion gap metabolic acidosis
- Diabetic ketoacidosis
- Uraemia/urate
- Paraldehyde
- Ethylene glycol
- Lactic acidosis
- Methanol
- Alcohol/acid ingestion
- Salicylates

Causes of *normal* anion gap metabolic acidosis
- Renal failure
- Diarrhoea
- Ureteric diversion (e.g. ileal loop)
- Addison's disease
- RTA
- Drugs (e.g. acetazolamide)
- Pancreatic fistula

Respiratory acidosis
On ABG: pH <7.35, pCO_2 raised, BE and HCO_3^- normal with a low pO_2 = Type 2 respiratory failure – *see Respiratory* section.

Metabolic alkalosis

On ABG: pH >7.45, BE > +2, HCO_3 > 26 mmol/L. Causes: profuse vomiting, over-dose of alkaline substance, low K^+.

Respiratory alkalosis

On ABG: pH >7.45, pCO_2 low, and pO_2 low = Type 1 respiratory failure – *see Respiratory* section.

5.7. Electrolyte abnormalities

Hyponatraemia = low serum sodium

Results in neurological compromise. Serum/urine osmolalities and urinary sodium will help guide diagnosis in hyponatraemia, e.g. if serum osmolality is low (i.e. blood is dilute) but urine is inappropriately concentrated, then diagnosis is SIADH. If urinary sodium is raised, then salt loss is via the kidneys, e.g. diuretic use.

Management of hyponatraemia

Salt Deficit (patients are dehydrated)
Slowly correct hyponatraemia with normal saline. If rapid correction of low serum sodium, then central pontine myelinosis may result with neurological compromise.

- Diuretics
- Diarrhoea/vomiting
- Fistula
- Addison's disease
- Burns

Excess Water retention
Correct management is with fluid restriction

- CCF
- Nephrotic syndrome
- SIADH
- Liver disease
- Hypothyroidism
- Psychogenic polydipsia

Hypernatraemia = high serum sodium

Causes: dehydration, e.g. diarrhoea or vomiting; diabetes insipidus. Treatment: rehydration (PO or IV).

Hyperkalaemia = high serum potassium

K^+ >6.5 mmol/L demands urgent treatment (*see Renal emergencies* below). Causes: acute/chronic renal failure, rhabdomyolysis, massive blood tranfusion, iatrogenic (infusion of IV fluid containing K), K-sparing diuretics, metabolic acidosis (*Note:* acidosis and hyperkalaemia are usually associated – exceptions to the rule include RTA type 1 and 2), drugs (e.g. ACE-inhibitors), Addison's disease.

Hypokalaemia = low serum potassium

Causes: can be due to either *renal losses* (e.g. diuretics, Cushing's syndrome, Conn's syndrome, renal tubular losses, Liddle's/Bartter's/Gitelman's syndrome) or *extrarenal losses* (e.g. vomiting, diarrhoea, alkalosis). Clinical features: weakness, lethargy, cramps. Investigations: ECG may demonstrate small/inverted T waves, U waves. Management: correct Mg^+ as well as K^+ (otherwise K^+ will be difficult to correct). With IV or PO supplementation depending on severity.

5.8. Renal emergencies and investigations

Hyperkalaemia

K^+ >6.5 mmol/L is associated with cardiac arrest and requires immediate action.

Investigations: ECG may demonstrate prolonged PR interval, tented T-waves, followed by broadening of the QRS complex and bradycardia/VF/PEA.

MANAGEMENT
- Place patient on cardiac monitor.
- Establish and eliminate cause of hyperkalaemia, e.g. ARF (needs dialysis?), ACE-inhibitor/ARB (withdrawal may bring K^+ down); CRF (low K^+ diet?).
- Drug treatment:
  - 10 ml 10% calcium gluconate IV (protects heart but does not alter serum K^+)
  - 10–15 units insulin in 50 ml 50% glucose – lowers serum K^+ temporarily by pushing K^+ into the cells. Monitor BM
  - salbutamol nebulisers – may not be effctive
  - consider IV sodium bicarbonate 1.26% if metabolic acidosis
  - calcium resonium can be used to control K^+ in the longer term but side effects (such as constipation) common and it is not usually recommended.

Renal investigations
URINE DIPSTICK (NEVER FORGET THE URINE)
Blood	=	UTI, ureteric stone, urothelial malignancy or inflammation (GN).
Protein	=	non-specific for a host of renal diseases. *Never ignore protein/blood on dip: it is never normal.*
Nitrites	=	UTI.
Leucocytes	=	UTI or interstitial nephritis.

URINE MICROSCOPY
Red cell casts	=	GN.
White cell casts	=	pyelonephritis, acute interstitial nephritis.
Granular casts	=	ATN.
Organisms	=	UTI – send for MC&S to identify organism type and sensitivity.

ULTRASOUND RENAL TRACT Indications: to exclude obstruction; to measure size of kidneys (unequal size = RVD, small = CRF) and assess structure (increased echogenicity indicates parenchymal disease, multiple cysts seen in APKD).

RENAL BIOPSY Indications: to aid diagnosis of significant renal disease or to establish prognosis. Generally appropriate if haematuria or proteinuria of unknown cause; deteriorating renal function of unknown cause; and to determine prognosis in certain cases. Complications: bleeding is the main risk and patients should be consented for this.

INSERTION OF CENTRAL VENOUS CATHETER Indications: fluid management and access for IV treatment. NICE guidelines recommend ultrasound-guided line insertion. Complications: bleeding, infection, pneumothorax, air embolus, failure of procedure.

6

Endocrinology and metabolism

6.1. Diabetes mellitus

Type 1: 10–15% of cases; insulin deficiency as a consequence of pancreatic β-cell destruction.

Type 2: 85–90% of cases; insulin resistance.

There are some disorders which can lead to 'secondary' diabetes mellitus:
- Pancreatic disease (e.g. pancreatitis, cancer, cystic fibrosis, haemochromatosis).
- Drugs (e.g. steroids).
- Other endocrine disorders (e.g. Cushing's, acromegaly).

Insulin deficiency or resistance has multiple metabolic sequelae with chronic hyperglycaemia being the major feature.

CLINICAL FEATURES   Patients may present acutely (most commonly in type 1 with DKA), or with more chronic symptoms (most commonly in type 2): polyuria (and polydipsia), weight loss, recurrent infections.

DIAGNOSIS   Fasting glucose ≥ 7 mmol/L or random glucose ≥ 11.1 mmol/L (on one occasion if symptomatic, or two occasions if asymptomatic). Some patients have 'prediabetes' or impaired glucose tolerance (IGT), defined as a glucose level between 7.8–11 mmol/L, two hours after a glucose load in the oral glucose tolerance test (OGTT).

Type 1 Diabetes Mellitus

The majority of patients are <18 years old at onset (about 60%) but it can present in adults. There is autoimmune destruction of β-cells. Antibodies present include those to islet cells; other autoimmune conditions may co-exist. Genetic risk factors include certain HLA associations (e.g. DR3/4). Environmental triggers are unclear.

Type 2 Diabetes Mellitus

Generally occurs in older patients (>40 years). Incidence is increasing as obesity and other risk factors also become more prevalent. Associated with the 'metabolic syndrome': insulin resistance with hypertension, hyperlipidaemia, obesity and microalbuminuria. Rarely, younger patients develop type 2 DM (maturity onset diabetes of the young or MODY) – due to mutations in genes such as glucokinase.

GENERAL MANAGEMENT

- Encourage self-monitoring of capillary blood glucose (CBG or 'BM').
- Monitor HbA1c – aim for levels of <7% in most cases.
- Screen for complications at regular intervals, i.e. retinopathy, nephropathy, neuropathy.
- Patient education – give advice regarding: diet; rotation of injections sites; insulin dosage in different circumstances, e.g. exercise, intercurrent illness; and how to treat hypo- and hyperglycaemia.

DRUG MANAGEMENT

- Type 1: insulin – intermittent subcutaneous injections (although some have pumps). Common regimes are 'basal-bolus' (single daily dose of a long-acting insulin with a short-acting insulin before each meal) or twice-daily mixed insulin (e.g. 30% short acting and 70% long acting).
- Type 2: stepped management:
  - Lifestyle change – healthy diet, exercise, weight loss.
  - Monotherapy – if overweight, metformin; if not, sulphonylurea, e.g. gliclazide. Consider a glitazone (e.g. pioglitazone).
  - Combination therapy – consider any combination of the above three types of drugs.
  - Insulin if inadequate glycaemic control on combination therapy.
  - GLP-1 (Glucagon-like peptide-1) analogues and DPP-IV (dipeptidyl peptidase-IV) inhibitors are now licensed.

Microvascular complications – the 'triopathy'

1. Retinopathy
   a) Background: microaneurysms, hard exudates, haemorrhages (dot, blot, flame).
   b) Pre-proliferative: cotton wool spots, venous abnormalities (dilation, beading).
   c) Proliferative: neovascularisation; and if advanced, vitreous haemorrhage, tractional retinal detachment and rubeotic glaucoma.
   d) Maculopathy: retinopathy within a disc width of the macula.

Management: ensure tight glycaemic and BP control; fibrates may have a role; monitor and detect retinopathy early; laser photocoagulation if proliferative or maculopathy.

2. Neuropathy
   a) *Peripheral neuropathy:* (mainly sensory) – glove/stocking sensory loss.
   b) *Painful neuropathy:* can be acute onset, e.g. with insulin therapy.
   c) *Mononeuropathy:* (limb/cranial) – may be due to entrapment (e.g. carpal tunnel syndrome) or infarction; multiple nerves can be involved ('mononeuritis multiplex').
   d) *Diabetic 'amyotrophy':* mainly seen with type 2 DM – typically asymmetric proximal lower limb weakness, wasting and pain with absent knee reflexes.
   e) *Autonomic neuropathy:* cardiovascular (e.g. postural hypotension), GI (e.g.

diarrhoea), and genitourinary (e.g. erectile dysfunction) involvement; other features include hypoglycaemic unawareness and sweating.

3. Nephropathy

Initially patients will have microalbuminuria (monitor urine albumin/creatinine ratio) and may then later develop overt proteinuria and chronic renal failure. Management: reduce proteinuria with ACE-inhibitors +/– angiotensin receptor blockers.

Macrovascular complications, i.e. ischaemic heart disease, peripheral vascular disease and cerebrovascular disease

Preventative measures include improving glycaemic control, smoking cessation, anti-platelet therapy, exercise, dietary advice and treatment of hypertension, reduction in microalbuminuria/proteinuria (ACE-inhibitors +/– angiotensin II receptor antagonists), obesity (e.g. orlistat) and hyperlipidaemia (e.g. statin).

The diabetic foot

Typically occurs as a result of peripheral vascular disease and/or neuropathy; may lead to ulcers +/– infections. Management requires avoidance of mechanical stress to the limb and a multi-disciplinary approach with referral to a diabetologist (for strict diabetic control), vascular surgeon (for improvement of blood supply to the limb, if indicated) and podiatrist.

Emergencies
Diabetic ketoacidosis (DKA)

Type 1 DM can present acutely as DKA (often as the first presentation). Triggers in known diabetics include poor compliance with insulin treatment and infection. Clinical features: dehydration, nausea and vomiting, abdominal pain, hyperventilation, drowsiness and decreased level of consciousness.

INVESTIGATIONS   Blood glucose is high (normally 7.1–20 mmol/l); ABG demonstrates a metabolic acidosis (plasma pH <7.30); blood ketones >1 mmol/l and urinalysis is also positive for ketones. Management: rehydration with intravenous fluids and an intravenous insulin infusion are necessary with close monitoring of plasma potassium.

Hyperosmolar non-ketotic diabetic coma (HONK)

Poorly controlled type 2 DM may lead to HONK. Precipitating factors: infection, drugs (e.g. steroids or thiazides) and MI.

CINICAL FEATURES   Patients may be very dehydrated, nauseous and drowsy with decreasing levels of consciousness as it becomes more severe.

INVESTIGATIONS   Blood glucose is very high (>30 mmol/l), and likewise plasma osmolality. However, there are no (or only a trace of) ketones and no (or only a mild) acidosis.

MANAGEMENT   Rehydration with intravenous fluids and an intravenous insulin infusion are necessary with close monitoring of plasma potassium. Patients are at risk of venous thromboses and therefore SC heparin should also be given.

Note: a subgroup of type 2 DM can present with ketotic-prone acidosis. The treatment is as above, and often the patient will need to remain on SC insulin for a short period to allow the pancreatic beta-cells to recover. They can eventually be treated with oral hypoglycaemics.

Hypoglycaemia

CLINICAL FEATURES   Initially autonomic symptoms – palpitations, sweating, hunger, anxiety, nausea. As hypoglycaemia becomes more severe, neuroglycopenic symptoms occur – confusion and altered consciousness, dizziness and if severe seizures.
- In patients with known DM, the cause is usually inadvertent excess insulin or hypoglycaemic drug use, e.g. with alcohol use, after altered diet or exercise.
- Other causes include (*mnemonic is DELTA*): **d**rugs (e.g. aspirin overdose), **e**ndocrine (e.g. insulinoma, Addison's, hypopituitarism), **l**iver disease, **t**umours (sarcoma, hepatoma) and **a**lcohol.

TREATMENT   In mild cases oral glucose (e.g. a sugary drink) will suffice but if severe, consider giving either IM glucagon or IV glucose, e.g. 50 ml 50% dextrose.

6.2. Pituitary and hypothalamic disease
Anterior pituitary
Dopamine release from the hypothalamus inhibits prolactin release while TRH, CRF, GnRH and GHRH stimulate release of their associated pituitary hormones:

HYPOTHALAMUS	PITUITARY	MAIN TARGET GLAND	HORMONES PRODUCED
TRH	TSH	Thyroid	T4/T3
CRF and AVP	ACTH	Adrenal cortex	Cortisol
GnRH	FSH/LH	Testes/ovaries	Testosterone/oestrogen
GHRH	GH	Liver	IGF-1
Dopamine inhibits (TRH stimulates)	Prolactin	Mammary glands	

Posterior pituitary
Antidiuretic hormone (arginine vasopressin or AVP) and oxytocin are synthesised in the supraoptic and paraventricular nuclei of the hypothalamus and stored and then finally secreted from the posterior pituitary. AVP acts on V2 receptors on the basolateral membrane of the distal nephron leading to water conservation.

Pituitary tumours
The majority are benign adenomas, which may be non-secreting or secrete excess amounts of hormone. Management: depends on type of tumour.

CLINICAL FEATURES
Hormonal effects
- Fewer hormones, i.e. hypopituitarism (*see* below).
- More hormones: prolactinomas (hyperprolactinaemia); GH (acromegaly); ACTH (Cushing's disease); TSH and GnRH secreting tumours are rare.

Local mass effects (due to pressure on adjacent structures)
- Bitemporal hemianopia (optic chiasm).
- Cavernous sinus syndrome.

Hypopituitarism

Often caused by pituitary tumours. Other causes include sarcoid, TB, autoimmune disease, Sheehan's syndrome and iatrogenic (e.g. surgery, radiation). Hormones are normally lost in a characteristic order (as below); prolactin is rarely affected:
- GH deficiency: dwarfism in children; but in adults – depression and effects on bone and muscle.
- LH/FSH deficiency (hypogonadism): in men – lower libido, impotence, loss of body hair, loss of sperm production; in women – amenorrhoea, decreased breast size, atrophy of the genitals.
- TSH deficiency: hypothyroidism.
- ACTH deficiency: loss of skin pigmentation, adrenal failure (*see* Addison's).

Management: hormone replacement with thyroxine, hydrocortisone, testosterone or oestrogen +/– GH. Note that large tumours may cause ADH deficiency, i.e. diabetes inspidius, and treatment is with a vasopressin analogue DDAVP (desmopressin).

Hyperprolactinaemia

Often caused by pituitary tumours but also dopamine antagonists (e.g. antipsychotics) and hypothyroidism. Clinical features depend on gender: in women (who present earlier) – amenorrhoea, infertility, galactorrhoea; in men – loss of libido, impotence, infertility, galactorrhoea. Management: if secondary to a prolactinoma, medical treatment initially with a dopamine agonist, consider trans-sphenoidal surgery should this fails.

Acromegaly

Excessive amounts of GH in adult life, normally due to a GH-secreting pituitary tumour. The classical physical appearance suggests the diagnosis.
- Enlarged hands and feet (increased ring/glove/shoe size).
- Coarsening of facial features (thickened skin, enlargement of the nose, enlargement of the mandible – prognathism – with spreading of the teeth).

Other features.
- Enlargement of the internal organs (e.g. cardiomyopathy).
- Diabetes mellitus and hypertension.
- Bitemporal hemianopia (due to pressure on the optic chiasm).
- Entrapment neuropathies (e.g. carpal tunnel syndrome).

Note: Before epiphyseal fusion, excess GH causes **gigantism**.

INVESTIGATIONS
- Raised IGF-1 used to screen for disease.
- Lack of suppression of GH levels with a glucose tolerance test (gold standard).
- MRI of the pituitary fossa.
- Formal assessment of visual fields.

MANAGEMENT Surgical: trans-sphenoidal hypophysectomy is first-line. Medical treatment includes dopamine agonists (e.g. bromocriptine, cabergoline), somatostatin analogues (octreotide, lanreotide) and GH receptor antagonists (pegvisomant). Radiotherapy is also an option.

Diabetes inspidus (DI)

CLINICAL FEATURES Polyuria + polydipsia. Two forms – cranial and nephrogenic:

- Cranial DI is caused by damage to the hypothalamus or posterior pituitary – with loss of ADH.
  - Causes: pituitary surgery, tumours, e.g. craniopharyngioma, sarcoid, trauma.
- Nephrogenic DI is caused by inability of ADH to act on the kidney.
  - Causes: diseases of the kidneys, hypercalcaemia, hypokalaemia, drugs, congenital.

DIAGNOSIS Made by measuring plasma and urine osmolalities during a water deprivation test, and following an injection of DDAVP (desmopressin – a synthetic version of ADH).

MANAGEMENT If nephrogenic, treat underlying cause; if cranial DI, consider DDAVP replacement.

6.3. Thyroid disease
TSH (produced from the anterior pituitary) stimulates T4 (thyroxine) and T3 (triiodothyronine) production from thyroid gland. T4 converted to active T3 in tissues by deiodinase.

Hyperthyroidism
Cause: most commonly due to thyroid disease, i.e. high T4/T3 with suppressed TSH. Only very rarely due to hypothalamic or pituitary disease (high TSH and high T4/T3). More common in women.

Causes of hyperthyroidism

○ Graves' disease	○ Toxic multinodular goitre (MNG)
○ Toxic adenoma	○ Thyroiditis (subacute, silent or post-partum)

CLINICAL FEATURES
- Weight loss and increased appetite.
- Fine postural tremor.
- Tachycardia and palpitations.
- Heat intolerance and sweating.
- Agitation and irritability.
- Diarrhoea.
- Others: proximal myopathy, lid lag/retraction, oligomenorrhoea, heart failure, AF.

Rarely, presents as an emergency (thyrotoxic crisis or thyroid storm) with anxiety, agitation, tachycardia, tremor +/– decreased consciousness and heart failure.

Graves' disease
Autoimmune disease. Features specific to Graves' disease (that do not occur with other causes):
- ○ Eye signs – exophthalmos, ophthalmoplegia, chemosis of the conjunctivae
- ○ Pretibial myxoedema
- ○ Thyroid acropachy

INVESTIGATIONS
- If primary: raised T4 and T3, suppressed TSH.
- TSH receptor antibody: positive in Graves'.

- Thyroid uptake scan: diffuse increased uptake in Graves', nodular uptake in MNG, no uptake in thyroiditis.

MANAGEMENT
- Medical
  - Propranolol may be symptomatically useful initially.
  - Antithyroid drugs (carbimazole, propylthiouracil): side effects of rash, joint pains, agranulocytosis. Propylthiouracil preferred in pregnancy.
  - Radioiodine: used first line for some patients with Graves' or toxic MNG, those who have relapsed after initial drug treatment or allergies to drug treatment.
- Surgery
  - Thyroidectomy – useful in large goitres, if relapse after initial drug treatment, or in patients with contraindications to the above treatments.

Hypothyroidism

Most commonly caused by primary thyroid disease, i.e. low T4/T3 with high TSH. Only very rarely is hypothalamic or pituitary disease a cause (low TSH and low T4/T3). More common in women.

Causes of hypothyroidism

- ○ Autoimmune
- ○ Iatrogenic: thyroidectomy, radioiodine, drugs, e.g. amiodarone, lithium
- ○ Hashimoto's thyroiditis
- ○ Iodine deficiency (common in developing countries)

CLINICAL FEATURES
- Weight gain.
- Skin problems: dry skin with myxoedema.
- Bradycardia.
- Cold intolerance.
- Fatigue and lethargy.
- Constipation.

Others: hoarse voice, psychiatric disorders (depression, dementia, and rarely psychosis), serous effusions (e.g. pleural, pericardial). Rarely, presents as an emergency (myxoedema coma) with hypothermia, hypoglycaemia, hypotension and decreased consciousness.

INVESTIGATIONS
- If primary: raised TSH, low T4 (normal T4 in subclinical hypothyroidism).
- FBC: possibly macrocytic anaemia.
- Thyroid autoantibodies (thyroid peroxidase and microsomal antibodies): may be positive in Hashimoto's.

TREATMENT Replacement with oral levothyroxine (T4).

Thyroid swellings/goitre

May be euthyroid, raised T4 or low T4. Causes:
- ○ Simple idiopathic goitre
- ○ Multinodular goitre
- ○ Autoimmune: Graves' disease, Hashimoto's
- ○ Others: thyroiditis, iodine deficiency, dyshormonogenesis, drugs

Thyroid cancer

Primary thyroid malignancies are rare and normally present as a euthyroid solitary nodule. Types of thyroid cancer: papillary (70%), follicular (20%), anaplastic (<5%). Medullary tumours are derived from the C-cells of the thyroid, rather than the epithelium – characteristically, these secrete calcitonin.

6.4. Adrenal disease

The adrenal gland consists of the cortex and medulla. Within the cortex there are three zones:

○ **zona glomerulosa:** produces mineralocorticoids – mainly aldosterone. Renin (from kidney) stimulates conversion of angiotensinogen (from liver) to angiotensin I, which is converted to angiotensin II in the lung by ACE. Angiotensin II stimulates aldosterone production

○ **zona fasciculata:** produces glucocorticoids – mainly cortisol. CRF/AVP stimulate ACTH production by the pituitary which stimulates cortisol production

○ **zona reticularis:** produces sex steroids

The medulla secretes catecholamines (adrenaline, noradrenaline) in response to various stimuli, e.g. stress, fear.

Cushing's syndrome

Excess cortisol. More common in women.

CAUSES

- Iatrogenic Cushing's – secondary to steroid treatment.
- Cushing's disease – secondary to an ACTH-producing pituitary adenoma.
- Ectopic ACTH production – by neuroendocrine tumours, particularly in lung.
- Adrenal Cushing's – secondary to adrenal adenomas (or rarely carcinomas).

CLINICAL FEATURES

- Fat redistribution: obesity (centripetal), buffalo hump, 'moon face'.
- Skin: thin skin, easy bruising, purple striae.
- Metabolic: hypertension, diabetes mellitus, recurrent infections, proximal myopathy, osteoporosis.
- Psychiatric problems: depression, psychosis.

INVESTIGATIONS

- Confirm raised cortisol with one or more of the following:
  - Absent diurnal variation in cortisol: should not be detectable at midnight but is detectable in endogenous Cushing's syndrome.
  - Raised 24 hour urinary cortisol excretion.
  - Failure to suppress cortisol during 48 hour low-dose dexamethasone suppression test.
- Establish cause.
  - Measure ACTH: very high in ectopic, raised in Cushing's disease, suppressed in adrenal causes.
  - 48 hour high-dose dexamethasone suppression test.
  - Imaging: adrenal CT, pituitary MRI, chest CT.
  - Rarely, other specialist tests necessary, e.g. petrosal sinus sampling.

MANAGEMENT   Cushing's disease is treated with pituitary surgery +/– radiotherapy. For ectopic ACTH secretion, treat underlying carcinoma, and if necessary use metyrapone +/– ketoconazole to control cortisol production. If necessary, both adrenals can be removed but beware Nelson's syndrome (uncontrolled growth of Cushing's disease tumour causing hyperpigmentation). Adrenal Cushing's is treated with surgery to remove tumour.

Conn's syndrome

Excess aldosterone – normally due to an adrenal adenoma (>75%) and less commonly, due to bilateral adrenal hyperplasia. Clinical features: hypertension and hypokalaemia (which causes muscle weakness and cramps, polyuria and polydipsia) and metabolic alkalosis.

MANAGEMENT
- Confirm diagnosis: plasma aldosterone (high) and renin (usually low).
- Establish cause: CT abdomen (occasionally adrenal venous sampling is required if tumour not seen on imaging).
- If adenoma confirmed, surgical excision. If bilateral adrenal hyperplasia, aldosterone receptor blockers (e.g. spironolactone) + other antihypertensives.

Adrenal failure

Primary adrenal failure (Addison's disease) is most often due to autoimmune adrenalitis (>70%). Rare causes include TB and CMV. Secondary failure is due to failure of ACTH production by the pituitary, either due to hypopituitarism or due to steroid suppression of the hypothalamic pituitary axis (HPA).

CLINICAL FEATURES   Often non-specific: lethargy, loss of appetite, weakness, weight loss. Other symptoms include abdominal pain and hyperpigmentation (particularly of oral mucosa). Biochemically there is low Na^+, high K^+ (in primary).

DIAGNOSIS   Short Synacthen test – demonstrates failure of plasma cortisol response to ACTH injection.

MANAGEMENT
- Lifelong steroid replacement with hydrocortisone and fludrocortisone is necessary (remember to give patient a steroid card and advice about increasing dose during illness).
- Occasionally, patients may present acutely with an Addisonian crisis (e.g. after haemorrhage or rapid withdrawal of longstanding steroid therapy) with hypovolaemia and hypotension. Treat with intravenous fluids and steroids.

Phaeochromocytoma and paragangliomas

A phaeochromocytoma is an adrenal medulla tumour. A paraganglioma is a tumour arising from the sympathetic and parasympathetic ganglia. ≈ 25% occur due to mutations in the VHL, NF1, c-Ret, SDH-B, -C, -D genes and are associated with familial phaeo/paraganglioma syndromes. Clinical features: classical symptoms are headache, sweating and palpitations, which may be paroxysmal, occurring in attacks lasting minutes to hours; and hypertension which may be persistent rather than episodic.

DIAGNOSIS   Raised urinary and plasma catecholamines or metanephrines.

MANAGEMENT
- Locate tumour: CT/MRI abdomen +/– MIBG scanning (may be useful to identify small tumours and particularly metastases).

- Treatment: initially alpha-blocker (e.g. phenoxybenzamine) and β-blocker (e.g. propranolol) are given to control hypertension. Followed by surgery to remove tumour.
- Consider genetic screening especially if family history or patient young (<40 years).

6.5. Parathyroid disease and calcium metabolism

Low calcium stimulates parathyroid hormone (PTH) release from the parathyroid gland. PTH causes reabsorption of calcium from bone and kidney, and stimulates hydroxylation of vitamin D to its active form (which in turn increases GI calcium reabsorption).

Hyperparathyroidism

- Primary – causes: adenoma or more rarely hyperplasia of the glands. Treatment is with parathyroidectomy.
- Secondary – caused in response to hypocalcaemia (*see* below).
- Tertiary – in longstanding secondary hyperparathyroidism PTH production becomes autonomous. Treatment is with parathyroidectomy.

Hypercalcaemia

Causes:
- Primary (and tertiary) hyperparathyroidism
- Myeloma
- Malignancy
- Sarcoidosis

The classic mnemonic for clinical features is 'bones, stones, groans and psychic moans', i.e. bone pain, renal stones, abdominal pain (with vomiting and constipation) and depression. Management: patients need to be rehydrated and the underlying cause treated. If necessary, intravenous bisphosphonates can be given.

Hypoparathyroidism

Most commonly follows thyroid or parathyroid surgery. Can be autoimmune.

Pseudohypoparathyroidism

PTH resistance due to abnormal PTH receptor. Clinical features: short, round face, short metacarpals, learning difficulties.

Pseudopseudohypoparathyroidism

Same clinical features as for pseudohypoparathyroidism but biochemistry is normal.

Hypocalcaemia

Causes:
- Chronic renal failure
- Hypoparathyroidism
- Vitamin D deficiency

Symptoms (if any) are mainly neurological (tetany, seizures) or psychiatric. Eponymous signs:
- Chvostek's sign – twitching of the facial muscles on tapping over the facial nerve
- Trousseau's sign – spasm of the hand and thumb following occlusion of the blood flow to the upper arm with a blood pressure cuff inflated to 10 mmHg above systolic BP for up to three minutes

Treatment: Oral calcium (IV if severe or symptomatic) combined with vitamin D in most circumstances.

Osteomalacia

Usually due to vitamin D deficiency, e.g. secondary to poor diet, GI disorders such as malabsorption, lack of sun exposure. Symptoms are bone and muscle pain, proximal myopathy and subclinical fractures. In childhood, vitamin D deficiency causes rickets with skeletal deformities, e.g. bowed legs. Treat underlying disorder and give vitamin D.

Paget's disease

○ Disease of abnormal bone turnover
○ Often asymptomatic and diagnosed from an isolated raised ALP
○ Clinical features if symptomatic: bone pain, overgrowth of bone leading to compressive neuropathies, e.g. VIII cranial nerve and deafness, deformities
○ Management: does not require treatment unless symptomatic

	CALCIUM	PHOSPHATE
Primary hyperparathyroidism	+	−
Secondary hyperparathyroidism	−	+
Tertiary hyperparathyroidism	+	− or +
Hypoparathyroidism	−	+
Osteomalacia	Normal or −	Normal or −
Osteoporosis	Normal	Normal

+ = raised, − = lowered

6.6. Multiple endocrine neoplasia (MEN)

Autosomal dominant syndromes associated with various tumours of the endocrine system.

MEN I: mutations in menin

● Parathyroid hyperplasia or adenoma – often the first diagnosed with hypercalcaemia.
● Pituitary – usually prolactinoma, more rarely secrete GH or ACTH.
● Pancreas – insulinoma or gastrinoma.

MEN IIA: mutations in c-Ret

● Medullary carcinoma of the thyroid.
● Phaeochromocytomas – usually multiple.
● Parathyroid hyperplasia or adenoma.

MEN IIB: mutations in c-Ret

● Medullary carcinoma of the thyroid.
● Marfanoid appearance.
● Mucosal ganglioneuromas around mouth + in intestine (can cause obstruction).
● Phaeochromocytomas.
● Parathyroid hyperplasia rare.

6.7. Lipid disorders

- Raised LDL cholesterol is associated with vascular disease (although HDL cholesterol is protective).
- Raised triglycerides also increase vascular risk.

Primary hyperlipidaemias

Include familial hypercholesterolaemia where there is LDL receptor dysfunction leading to raised LDL (and total) cholesterol. Clinical features: myocardial infarctions occur at young age; tendon xanthomas and xanthelasma may be present.

Secondary hyperlipidaemia

Causes include alcohol, chronic liver disease and chronic renal failure.

Drugs that lower lipid levels

- Statins (e.g. simvastatin, atorvastatin) are HMG-CoA reductase inhibitors and inhibit liver synthesis of cholesterol. Side effects: myositis (rare)
- Fibrates (e.g. bezafibrate) are PPAR-alpha agonists
- Ezetimibe and plant sterols inhibit cholesterol absorption in the intestine
- Nicotinic acid

6.8. Porphyria

A group of rare disorders caused by abnormalities of the enzymes in the haem synthesis pathway. Two are more commonly encountered compared to others.

Acute intermittent porphyria

Autosomal dominant condition. Often onset is in teens to twenties. Clinical features: GI symptoms (abdominal pain, constipation) with neuropsychiatric problems (including seizures) and neuropathy. Often symptoms are episodic – precipitated by various drugs including alcohol. Investigations: urine turns dark red on standing.

Porphyria cutanea tarda

Often sporadic in association with chronic liver disease (commonly alcohol-related). Clinical features: photosensitive rash. Investigations: urine normal in colour.

7

Rheumatology

7.1. Rheumatoid arthritis (RA)

Chronic, symmetrical inflammatory polyarthropathy that can be deforming. Incidence: 3:1 male to female ratio; onset commonly between 40–50 years.

CLINICAL FEATURES Joints
- Pain: worse in the morning.
- Stiffness: worse in the morning, relieved by activity.
- Swelling, warmth and tenderness in the affected joints when disease active (although may be masked due to use of NSAIDs).
- Symmetrical involvement of the MCP/PIP joints and wrist most commonly (although any synovial joint can be affected in RA) – classic features:
  - 'swan-neck' and Boutonnière deformities
  - 'z-shaped' thumb
  - ulnar deviation of the fingers.

In Rheumatoid Factor positive disease, rheumatoid nodules may be present – these typically overly the extensor surfaces, most commonly the elbow (and rarely lung).
RA is a multisystem disorder (*mnemonic – FRANCE-V*):
- **F**elty's syndrome: with splenomegaly and neutropenia.
- **R**espiratory: pleural disease, pulmonary fibrosis, pulmonary nodules.
- **A**myloidosis (secondary): may cause renal disease (rarely).
- **N**eurological: peripheral neuropathy or mononeuritis multiplex, carpal tunnel syndrome, cervical myelopathy due to atlanto-axial subluxation.
- **C**ardiac: pericardial disease.

- Eye: dry eyes (if Sjögren's), episcleritis, scleritis, rarely scleromalacia perforans.
- Vasculopathy (and rarely vasculitis): nail fold infarcts.

Early treatment (particularly with newer drugs) decreases the frequency of systemic complications.

INVESTIGATIONS
- Blood tests: anaemia can occur for many reasons, although most commonly it is an 'anaemia of chronic disease'.
- ESR/CRP – raised in active disease.
- Rheumatoid factor – positive in ≈ 70%.

MANAGEMENT
- Requires a multidisciplinary team approach, involve particularly physiotherapists and OT.
- Drugs therapy:
  - analgesia: paracetamol, opiates
  - NSAIDs
  - steroids: intra-articular, intramuscular, oral (usually only short term)
  - disease-modifying anti-rheumatic drugs (DMARDs): commonly methotrexate (others include gold, azathioprine, sulphasalazine)
  - anti-TNF therapy: e.g. infliximab, etanercept
  - rituximab.
- Surgery: may occasionally be necessary, e.g. joint replacement.

7.2. Seronegative arthritis
'Seronegative' means that the rheumatoid factor is negative.

Ankylosing spondylitis
Associated with HLA-B27 in ≈ 90% of cases; 5:1 male to female ratio; onset commonly between 20–40 years.

CLINICAL FEATURES
- Sacroiliitis and spondylitis.
  - Pain and stiffness, usually more marked in lower back.
  - Decreased movement in the spine and reduced chest expansion with classic stooped 'question-mark' posture and protruding abdomen.
- Peripheral arthritis (in 30–40%): commonly asymmetrical, affecting large-joints.
- Achilles tendonitis or other tenosynovitis.
- Other features (*mnemonic – A's*): **a**ortic regurgitation, **A**V block and other cardiac conduction abnormalities, **a**nterior uveitis, **a**pical lung fibrosis, **a**myloidosis, **a**tlanto-axial subluxation.

INVESTIGATIONS AND MANAGEMENT
- Spine x-ray: characteristic features of 'bamboo spine', syndesmophytes and loss of the lumbar lordosis.
- Multidisciplinary team approach (including physiotherapy), NSAIDs, anti-TNF.

Psoriatic arthropathy (*see also Dermatology section*)
Can occur with little skin involvement. There may be nail changes – pitting, onycholysis, hyperkeratosis. Five main forms:

- Symmetrical polyarthritis: 'RA'-like.
- DIP joints: 'OA'-like.
- Axial disease (sacroiliitis/spondylitis): 'Ankylosing spondylitis'-like.
- Asymmetrical oligoarthritis: 'Reiter's'-like.
- Arthritis mutilans (with 'telescoping' of the fingers).

MANAGEMENT   Analgesia, NSAIDs and disease modifying agents.

Reiter's syndrome/reactive arthritis
Triad of arthritis (asymmetrical, large joints), conjunctivitis and urethritis. Occurs after Chlamydia infection or less commonly a gastrointestinal infection.

Arthritis associated with inflammatory bowel disease
Can occur prior to the onset of IBD. Clinical features: most commonly an asymmetrical, large joint arthritis.

7.3. Crystal arthropathies
Gout
Caused by increased uric acid (although this is common and can be asymptomatic).

Causes of hyperuricaemia:
- *decreased uric acid excretion* – idiopathic (majority of cases), drugs (e.g. thiazides, ciclosporin), renal failure, alcohol
- *increased uric acid production* – rare genetic disorders (e.g. Lesch-Nyhan syndrome) or any cause of high cell turnover (e.g. myelo- and lymphoproliferative disorders, psoriasis).

Acute gout
Often monoarticular at presentation – first metatarsophalangeal joint most commonly affected. Joints are red, hot, swollen and very tender. Overlying skin may appear shiny and tight.

Chronic tophaceous gout
Chronically, gout may become polyarticular. Tophi = collections of uric acid crystals in the soft tissues may be present – ears, elbows and fingers are the most common sites.

INVESTIGATIONS   Negatively birefringent, needle-shaped crystals may be seen under polarised light. Treatment: NSAIDs or colchicine for acute attacks. Allopurinol for prevention of further attacks.

Pseudogout (calcium pyrophosphate deposition disease)
Clinical features: commonly asymptomatic with only radiological evidence of disease (chondrocalcinosis) but may present as:
- acute mono- or oligoarthritis: commonly knee or wrist
- secondary osteoarthritis: can affect many joints including MCP joints (rare in primary OA)
- similar to RA.

INVESTIGATIONS   Deposition of calcium pyrophosphate with positively birefringent rhomboid-shaped crystals seen under polarised light.

7.4. Septic arthritis

A *medical emergency.* Aetiology: in normal joints the most common cause is *Staph. aureus.* However, in young adults gonococcus is a common cause. Coagulase-negative *Staph.* causes septic arthritis in prosthetic joints. Other causes are *Haemophilus influenzae,* various *Strep.* species and Gram negative rods, although these are all more common in the very young.

CLINICAL FEATURES   An acutely red hot, swollen joint.

INVESTIGATIONS   It is important that the joint is aspirated and fluid sent for microscopy (including Gram stain) and culture as well as to look for crystals (the differential diagnosis includes gout/pseudogout).

MANAGEMENT   A prolonged course (6–12 weeks) of antibiotics (guided by culture and sensitivity) +/– surgical drainage and washout.

7.5. Osteoarthritis

Joint disease with initial loss of cartilage and secondary bone changes. Commonest form of arthritis. Incidence increases with increasing with age.

CLINICAL FEATURES   Involvement of one or two large weight-bearing joints is common, e.g. the hips or knees; spine is also commonly affected although any joint can be involved.

JOINTS FEATURES
- Pain.
- Stiffness – worse after activity.
- Instability of the joint with loss of function.
- Crepitus on moving the joint.
- Deformity/osteophytes as disease progresses.

Some patients will present with 'nodal' OA affecting the hands (PIP/DIP/first carpometacarpal joint *but rarely MCP in primary OA*): there are firm nodular swellings over the joints – Bouchard's nodes (PIP joints) and Heberden's nodes (DIP joints). Although the majority of cases are primary OA, there may be a secondary cause: other joint diseases (e.g. RA, septic arthritis, gout), metabolic disorders (e.g. haemochromatosis), and previous injury of the joint, congenital dysplastic disorders.

INVESTIGATIONS AND MANAGEMENT
- X-ray: characteristic appearance with loss of joint space, osteophytes, subchondral sclerosis, bone cysts.
- Conservative measures: appropriate footwear, weight loss, exercise, supportive aids.
- Analgesia.
- Surgery (e.g. joint replacement).

7.6. Osteoporosis

Loss of bone density, associated with an increased risk of fracture. May be primary or secondary, e.g. associated with steroid use.

CLINICAL FEATURES   May be asymptomatic. Often diagnosed following a fracture.

When osteoporosis affects the back there may be a decrease in height with progressive kyphosis secondary to vertebral collapse.

INVESTIGATIONS AND MANAGEMENT
- Imaging: dual energy x-ray absorptiometry (DEXA) scan.
- Calcium/vitamin D supplementation and a bisphosphonate commonly used to prevent further fracture or prevent fractures in those with risk factors.
- Other treatments: raloxifene (used in women where bisphosphonates are contraindicated) and teriparitide.

7.7. Systemic lupus erythematosus (SLE)

A multisystem autoimmune disorder of unknown aetiology. 10:1 female to male ratio.

CLINICAL FEATURES
- Arthralgia or arthritis.
- Rash.
- Malar ('butterfly').
- Discoid.
- Photosensitive.
- General systemic: fatigue, fever, lymphadenopathy.
- Haematological: anaemia (often haemolytic), thrombocytopenia, leucopenia.
- Ulcers: mouth.
- Neuropsychiatric: seizures, psychosis.
- Kidney: class I-V lupus nephritis.
- Serositis: pleuritis, pericarditis.

ANTIBODIES/OTHER BLOOD TESTS
- ANA: positive in > 95%.
- Anti-dsDNA: positive in ≈ 60% but specific.
- Anti-Sm: only positive in ≈ 20% but specific.
- Raised ESR with normal CRP (but CRP raised in infection/serositis/arthritis).
- Low complement: C3/C4.

MANAGEMENT
- Conservative measures: e.g. sunscreen/avoidance of sun if photosensitive rash.
- Hydroxychloroquine.
- Steroids.
- For renal disease: steroids +/– second agent depending on class (e.g. mycofenolate mofetil).
- Rituximab.

7.8. Antiphospholipid syndrome

CLINICAL FEATURES
- Arterial *and* venous thromboses (e.g. DVT, stroke/TIA).
- Recurrent miscarriages.
- Thrombocytopenia.
- Livedo reticularis.
- Migraine.

ANTIBODIES
- One or more are positive: anti-cardiolipin, false-positive VDRL test, anti-β_2-glycoprotein I, positive 'lupus anticoagulant'.

MANAGEMENT
- Optimise/eliminate risk factors, e.g. stop OCP, control BP, encourage smoking cessation.
- If evidence of thrombosis (may be venous of arterial) anticoagulate with initially SC heparin then warfarin.
- Counsel with regard to pregnancy.
- In select cases, further treatment may include plasma exchange, corticosteroids, IV immunoglobulin and cyclophosphamide.

7.9. Systemic sclerosis

A multisystem connective tissue disorder with fibrotic and vascular changes. First symptom (often years before others) is generally Raynaud's phenomenon. 5:1 female to male ratio. Classically divided into two categories: limited and diffuse, however, there is an overlap. Clinical features correlate with the pattern of autoantibodies present.

Limited systemic sclerosis
- Scleroderma (thickened skin) limited to face (beaked nose, microstomia), neck and the limbs distal to the elbow/knee.
- Formerly known as the CREST syndrome due to some of the features seen: Calcinosis, Raynaud's phenomenon, oEsophageal disease (reflux, dysmotility), Sclerodactyly, Telangiectasia.
- Pulmonary hypertension.

Diffuse systemic sclerosis
- Skin: scleroderma which can extend proximally to the elbow/knee and also to the face/trunk.
- Lungs: pulmonary fibrosis.
- Kidneys: renal crisis.
- Gastrointestinal (any part of gut): bacterial overgrowth, constipation.
- Cardiac: cardiomyopathy, arrhythmias.
- Musculoskeletal: arthralgia or more rarely arthritis, myositis.

Note: Localised form of disease with patches of scleroderma = morphoea.

ANTIBODIES
- ANA: positive in ≈ 90% of cases.
- Anti-centromere: classically seen in limited.
- Anti-Scl-70 (topoisomerase): classically seen in diffuse.
- Others: anti-RNA polymerase, anti-U3RNP.

MANAGEMENT
- Raynaud's: simple measures to keep hands warm, vasodilators (calcium-channel blockers) and if severe prostacyclin.
- Skin: methotrexate, cyclophosphamide and mycofenolate mofetil are all used.
- Renal: ACE-inhibitors (used in prevention/treatment of a renal crisis), prostacyclin.
- Pulmonary fibrosis: cyclophosphamide, steroids.
- Pulmonary HT: symptomatic treatment (e.g. diuretics), warfarin, prostacyclin, bosentan.
- Oesophageal: proton-pump inhibitors.

7.10. Sjögren's syndrome

An autoimmune disease causing lymphocytic infiltration of the exocrine glands (predominantly lacrimal and salivary glands). Occurs either as a primary disorder or with another connective tissue disease (secondary).

CLINICAL FEATURES

- Decreased secretion from exocrine glands:
  - dry eyes (positive Schirmer's test)
  - dry mouth.
- Systemic features can occur: Raynaud's phenomenon, fatigue, arthralgia/ arthritis, skin (e.g. purpura), peripheral neuropathy as well as respiratory, renal and liver involvement.
- Complications: increased incidence of lymphoma, particularly if anti-Ro or anti-La positive.

ANTIBODIES

- ANA.
- Anti-Ro or anti-La (positive in ≈ 60%).

MANAGEMENT

- Treat symptomatically:
  - dry eyes: artificial tears
  - dry mouth: saliva substitutes
  - systemic features: steroids/immunosuppresants.

7.11. Mixed connective tissue disease (MCTD)

There are patients who present with 'overlap syndromes' – features of different connective tissue diseases. In MCTD there are features of SLE, systemic sclerosis and polymyositis with positive anti-U1RNP antibodies:

- Raynaud's syndrome, swollen hands, sclerodactyly, arthritis, polymyositis and pulmonary fibrosis.

7.12. Autoantibodies

Autoantibodies of clinical significance

- ○ Rheumatoid factor (RF): antibody against IgG – seen in RA, cryoglobulinaemia
- ○ Anti-nuclear antibodies (ANA): seen in SLE, systemic sclerosis, Sjögren's syndrome, MCTD, polymyositis
- ○ Anti-double stranded DNA: seen in SLE
- ○ ENA (extractable nuclear antigens): anti-Ro, anti-La, anti-Sm, anti-centromere, anti-Jo1, anti-Scl70 (topoisomerase), anti-U1RNP, anti-RNA polymerase
- ○ Anti-neutrophil cytoplasmic antibodies (ANCA): p-ANCA (anti-MPO); c-ANCA (anti-PR3) – seen in vasculitis
- ○ Anti-phospholipid antibodies: anti-cardiolipin, anti-β_2-glycoprotein I, positive 'lupus anticoagulant'

7.13. Vasculitis

A group of heterogeneous conditions that feature inflammation of the blood vessel walls. Can be primary or can occur as part of another condition (secondary). Clinical features: initial symptoms of a systemic vasculitis are often non-specific – general malaise, fever, weight loss. Management: varies slightly for each type but generally steroids +/– immunosuppresants (e.g. cyclophosphamide).

Secondary
Vasculitis secondary to connective tissue disorders (SLE, Sjögren's, RA), infection, drug-induced, paraneoplastic.

Primary
Generally classified according to the size of the vessel predominantly affected, although there is overlap.

Large vessel
- **Giant cell arteritis (temporal arteritis)**
  Clinical features: headache with tenderness over temporal area; may have jaw claudication; sudden visual loss can occur secondary to an anterior ischaemic optic neuropathy. Management: needs urgent steroid treatment. Associated with polymyalgia rheumatica: proximal limb/shoulder muscle pain and stiffness (commonly morning) without weakness.
- **Takayasu's arteritis**
  Clinical features: claudication in arms, absent pulses, bruits.

Medium vessel
- **Polyarteritis nodosa**
  Can be associated with hepatitis B. Clinical features: microaneurysms with skin, kidney and gut involvement; mononeuritis multiplex.
- **Kawasaki disease**
  Mainly affects children. Clinical features: skin involvement (palms/soles) with coronary aneurysm formation and rarely myocardial infarcts.

Small vessel vasculitis
a) ANCA-associated – *measure antibody titres (c-ANCA = PR3 titre, p-ANCA = MPO titre)*
- **Wegener's granulomatosis:** c-ANCA positive in ≈ 90%; involvement of:
  1) sinuses, ears, eyes; 2) lungs (nodules, lung haemorrhage); 3) renal (glomerulonephritis).
- **Churg-Strauss syndrome:** p-ANCA positive in ≈ 70%; associated with asthma and eosinophilia.

b) Not-ANCA associated
- **Henoch-Schönlein purpura:** mainly affects children and generally self-limiting; palpable purpura over lower limbs/buttocks, arthralgia, abdominal pain and an IgA glomerulonephritis with haematuria.
- **Cryoglobulinaemia:** can be associated with hepatitis C.

Behçet's disease
Clinical features: orogenital ulceration, skin involvement including erythema nodosum and pathergy reaction, uveitis, venous thromboses, arthritis, neurological and GI involvement.

7.14. Collagen disorders
These heritable disorders of connective tissue (HDCT) are associated with joint hypermobility which is scored with the Beighton score (out of 9).
- Ability to put hands flat on the floor with knees straight (1).
- Hyperextension of the elbow beyond 90 degrees (1 for each side).
- Apposition of the thumb to the flexor aspect of the forearm (1 for each side).
- Hyperextension of the knee beyond 90 degrees (1 for each side).

● Passive dorsiflexion of the MCP joint to 90 degrees (1 for each side).

Marfan's syndrome
Autosomal dominant disorder with mutations in the fibrillin-1 gene.

CLINICAL FEATURES
● Marfanoid habitus: tall stature with long limbs (arm-span to height ratio >1.03), arachnodactyly (positive 'wrist' and 'thumb' signs), scoliosis, pectus carinatum or excavatum.
● Aortic dilatation: can lead to aortic regurgitation or dissection.
● High-arched palate.
● Lens dislocation.
● Joint hypermobility.
● Spontaneous pneumothoraces.

Osteogenesis imperfecta
A number of types which vary in severity.

CLINICAL FEATURES
● Bone fragility ('brittle bones') leading to multiple fractures.
● Blue sclerae.
● Short stature.
● Hearing problems.
● Joint hypermobility.

Ehlers-Danlos syndromes
A group of heterogeneous conditions (both clinically and genetically) with:
● Skin hyperextensibility.
● Fragile skin, delayed wound healing, atrophic scarring.
● Easy bruising.
● Joint hypermobility.

(Benign) joint hypermobility syndrome
CLINICAL FEATURES
● Joint hypermobility.
● Arthralgia.
● Often have mild features of other syndromes (e.g. marfanoid habitus, skin hyperextensibility).

8

Dermatology

8.1. Rashes

When describing a rash it is important to think about the following:

- Site: e.g. extensor surfaces (psoriasis), flexor surfaces (atopic eczema).
- Size and type:
  - macule – flat area of change in skin colour
  - patch – sometimes used to mean a macule greater than 1 cm
  - papule – raised lesion less than 1 cm
  - plaque – raised, flat-surfaced, disc-shaped lesion greater than 1 cm
  - nodule – raised solid, palpable lesion greater than 1 cm
  - vesicle – collection of fluid less than 1 cm
  - bulla – collection of fluid greater than 1 cm
  - pustule – collection of pus.
- Shape: e.g. round, linear or irregular.
- Sides (the border): well- or ill-defined.
- Surface: e.g. crust (dried exudate), lichenification (thickening of the skin).

8.2. Skin infections

Bacterial infections

- **Impetigo:** superficial skin infection caused by *Staph. aureus* or *Strep. pyogenes*. Clinical features: multiple lesions that may be vesicles, bullae or pustules. Normally a characteristic golden-coloured crust. Treatment: if localised, topical antibiotics can be used but in most cases systemic antibiotics (e.g. flucloxacillin) are required.
- **Cellulitis:** deep infection of the skin and subcutaneous tissues caused by *Strep. pyogenes* or *Staph. aureus*. Clinical features: skin becomes hot, red, tender and swollen. Edge is poorly defined. Patient may become systemically unwell with

fever. Treatment: if mild, oral antibiotics (e.g. penicillin V and flucloxacillin); if more severe, IV flucloxacillin and benzylpenicillin.
- **Folliculitis:** infection of the hair follicles, normally with *Staph. aureus*.

Viral infections
- **Herpes infections (simplex/zoster):** *see Infectious Disease section.*
- **Human papilloma virus (HPV) infection.**

CLINICAL FEATURES   Causes warts, i.e. raised lesions usually 1–2 cm in diameter – normally on hands or feet. Treatment: topical treatments (e.g. salicylic acid) or cryotherapy if resistant.
- **Others:** molluscum contagiosum; hand, foot and mouth disease.

Fungal infections – *see Infectious Disease section*

Infestations
Includes scabies (caused by *Sarcoptes scabiei*). Clinical features: pruritus, papular rash, burrows around hands/feet (often in finger web spaces). Treatment: permethrin or malathion; if lice (various types), malathion.

8.3. Eczema
Eczema = dermatitis, an inflammatory skin condition.

CLINICAL FEATURES
- Itching.
- Redness.
- Scaling.
- Papulovesicular rash.
- If chronic, the skin becomes thickened (lichenification).
- Can get secondary infection.

Atopic
Associated with other atopic diseases – asthma, hay fever. May appear in first year of life. Classically occurs in adulthood over flexures. Management: emollients and topical steroids.

Seborrhoeic
Associated with *Pitysporum* fungal infection. Clinical features: affects scalp, face, flexures. Often a scaly erythematous rash, particularly around nasolabial folds/ forehead. Treatment: topical ketoconazole (shampoo, cream) may be useful.

Contact
Delayed hypersensitivity to external allergens, e.g. nickel in jewellery. Can do patch testing if cause unclear. Treatment: acutely with topical steroids; remove/avoid allergen to prevent recurrence.

8.4. Acne vulgaris
Very common in adolescence with variable severity, although occasionally occurs in infants or in 30s/40s (mainly women). Skin lesions include:
- Comedones ('whiteheads' and 'blackheads').
- Papules, pustules, nodules.
- Later on there can be scarring.

TREATMENT
- Topical if mild disease: benzoyl peroxide, retinoic acid.
- Systemic: tetracycline or (in women) cyproterone acetate (Dianette) for moderate disease; isotretinoin for more severe disease (give advice regarding contraception and alcohol avoidance).

Rosacea
Often called 'acne rosacea' because lesions resemble acne (i.e. papules and pustules BUT *no comedones*). Most common in middle-aged women, over cheeks, forehead, nose, chin. Treatment: oral tetracyclines can be useful.

8.5. Skin tumours
Benign tumours
Seborrhoeic keratoses
Raised, flat, frequently pigmented lesions that typically develop on the trunk of the elderly. Extremely common and often multiple. They are often said to seem as if they are 'stuck-on'. Management: generally do not require treatment but can use cryotherapy.

Dermatofibroma
Small, asymptomatic firm papules, found mainly on the legs and more common in women.

Solar (actinic) keratoses
Erythematous, scaly patches found on light-exposed skin and caused by sun damage. Importantly, they are pre-malignant.

Malignant tumours
Basal cell carcinoma (BCC)
Occur on sun-exposed areas, particularly head and neck, in older people. Initially a pearly-white nodule with telangiectatic vessels on the surface which bleed easily. Later, expands outwards to leave a rolled edge with central ulceration (commonly then known as a 'rodent ulcer'). Locally invasive but rarely metastasises. Treatment: surgical excision +/- local radiotherapy. If superficial, curettage or cryotherapy may suffice.

Squamous cell carcinoma (SCC)
Occasionally remains confined to the epidermis, when it is known as SCC in situ or Bowen's disease. However, can be locally invasive and can metastasise to local lymph nodes. Related to sun exposure (therefore occurs on sun-exposed regions) but other factors are involved (e.g. smoking is associated with SCC of mouth/lips). Commonly presents as an ulcerated nodule but can present in other forms, e.g. a polypoid mass. Treatment: surgical excision +/- radiotherapy.

Malignant melanoma
Occurs in younger people than BCC or SCC but again related to sun exposure. Three main types:
- *superficial spreading:* (most common) pigmented macule or patch; irregular border and may have irregular pigmentation; may bleed or itch
- *nodular*
- *acral* (occur on sole or palm).

Malignant melanoma may also occur within a lentigo maligna. Prognosis depends on how deep the tumour is – the 'Breslow thickness' at biopsy. Treatment: surgical excision. Radiotherapy and chemotherapy are of little value.

Keratoacanthoma
Rapidly growing lump (over a couple of months) with central keratin-filled crater. Spontaneously resolves within 2–3 months leaving a scar. Recognition of this benign lesion is important as it can clinically (and histologically) resemble a squamous cell carcinoma, making it difficult to distinguish.

8.6. Psoriasis
Inflammatory disorder with hyperproliferation of epidermis. Occurs in ≈ 1% of the population in the developed world, of which one-third will have a family history (without any clear pattern of inheritance). Several clinical variants, e.g. classic plaque, pustular, guttate, erythrodermic.

CLINICAL FEATURES OF CLASSIC PLAQUE PSORIASIS
- Commonly affects the extensor surfaces (particularly knees and elbows) and the scalp.
- Single or multiple plaques which are silvery-red and scaly.
- Koebner phenomenon: lesions occur at sites of trauma/scarring.
- Nails may be affected: pitting, onycholysis.
- Arthritis – *see Rheumatology* section.

MANAGEMENT
- Topical: e.g. coal tar, dithranol, calcipotriol (vitamin D analogue).
- Systemic: e.g. methotrexate, acitretin, ciclosporin.
- Phototherapy: PUVA with oral psoralen.

8.7. Bullous disorders

Causes of vesicles/bullae
- ○ Infections (e.g. impetigo)
- ○ Insect bites
- ○ Drugs (e.g. barbiturates)
- ○ Metabolic disease (e.g. porphyria cutanea tarda)
- ○ Congenital disorders (e.g. epidermolysis bullosa)
- ○ Inflammatory disease (e.g. pemphigus, pemphigoid)

Pemphigus vulgaris
Superficial (epidermal) bullae which break easily causing erosions – lesions can be anywhere but commonly occur around the mouth. Positive Nikolsky sign (superficial skin layers slide off when pressure applied to 'normal' epidermis). Lesions can become secondarily infected. Treatment: high dose oral steroids followed by steroid-sparing agents.

Bullous pemphigoid
More common than pemphigus, usually occurring in the over-60s. Bullae are subepidermal, tense, and can occur anywhere but normally on the limbs (cf. cicatricial pemphigoid which commonly affects the mouth). Treatment: steroids or other immunosuppressive agents.

8.8. Naevi

Cutaneous hamartomas – commonest variety is the melanocytic naevus, i.e. collections of melanocytes; more commonly known as a 'mole'. Can be congenital or acquired (appear after birth). Pathologically, they begin as 'junctional' type (melanocytes collect at the dermoepidermal junction), and progress through two other stages ('compound', when cells migrate to the dermis and 'intradermal', when all cells are in the dermis). Clinical features: pigmented initially but may become pale later on when intradermal.

There is a small risk of malignant transformation (but note that the majority of melanomas do not arise in pre-existing naevi). Treatment: removal indicated if suspicion of malignant transformation, or for cosmetic reasons.

8.9. Erythroderma

Describes the situation where most of the skin becomes red.

CAUSES
- Psoriasis.
- Eczema.
- Mycosis fungoides/Sézary syndrome.
- Secondary to drugs.

COMPLICATIONS
- Abnormal control of temperature, e.g. hypothermia.
- Hypoalbuminaemia and peripheral oedema.
- Loss of water through the skin may lead to hypovolaemia.
- High-output cardiac failure.
- Sepsis.

Should be regarded as a *medical emergency*. Fluid resuscitation and treatment of the underlying cause and complications are required.

8.10. Other skin conditions
Erythema multiforme

Ranges from mild rash with the classic 'target' lesions over palms/soles, through to severe rash with inflammation also affecting mucous membranes, i.e. mouth, genitals and conjunctivae (when it is known as Stevens-Johnson syndrome). Triggered by infections (particularly herpes simplex), connective tissue disorders and a number of different drugs.

Pityriasis rosea

Normally starts with a 'herald' patch followed by pinkish patches with a scale around the edge, commonly over the trunk and said to be in the distribution of an inverted Christmas tree. Lesions also occur proximally on the limbs. Self-limiting.

8.11. Miscellaneous lesions
Lipoma

Common, slow-growing benign tumour of mature fat cells. Can occur in any location; usually found on the head and neck. Typically presents as a soft, fluctuant, lobulated mass which slips between the fingers ('slippage sign'). Can be multiple and may grow to a large size. Management: often excised for cosmesis or diagnosis.

Epidermoid cyst ('sebaceous cyst')

Common. Occurs due to a proliferation of epidermal cells within the dermis. Typically, slow-growing, occuring on the face, trunk, neck and scalp; solitary, firm, round and well-circumscribed, with a smooth surface and central punctum. Can be complicated by recurrent infections requiring antibiotics +/– incision and drainage acutely, followed by formal excision.

Dermoid cyst (Inclusion dermoid)

Uncommon. Painless, soft, smooth and slow growing. Can be classified as:
- **Congenital:** due to inclusion of the epidermis along lines of fusion of the skin dermatomes during embryological development. Usually presents in the face, neck or scalp at birth. Can produce symptoms due to external compression.
- **Acquired:** due to forced implantation of the epidermis into the dermis, e.g. in gardeners.

MANAGEMENT   Both types can be treated conservatively or surgically excised, if symptomatic.

Keloid scar

Abnormal scar formation due to excessive collagen production and/or decreased degradation. Scars typically extend beyond the wound margin. Usually affect the earlobes, chin, neck, shoulder and chest. Incidence is greater amongst black population (suggests racial predilection) and females with a peak age of presentation between 10 to 30 years. Scars are associated with burns, surgery, tattoos, injections, and bites, and tend to grow with time, puberty and pregnancy. Management: treat conservatively, due to inevitable recurrence with excision.

Hypertrophic scar

Unlike keloid scars these are confined to the wound margin and usually regress with time. They typically occur along flexor surfaces and skin creases and have no racial, age or gender predeliction. Management: surgical excision carries a high risk of recurrence, therefore treat conservatively.

Neurofibroma

Benign tumour of peripheral nerve elements. Lesions can be solitary or multiple and are typically pedunculated and nodular. Association with *café au lait* spots (>6) suggests Von Recklinghausen's disease (Neurofibromatosis type I), an autosomal dominant disorder associated with chromosome 17. Management: excision of lesions is indicated if painful.

Infectious disease

9.1. Bacterial infections

Gram-positive cocci
○ *Staphylococcus*
○ *Streptococcus*

Gram-positive rods
○ *Corynebacterium*
○ *Listeria*
○ *Bacillus*
○ Anaerobes, e.g. *Clostridium, Nocardia, Actinomyces*

Gram-negative cocci
○ *Neisseria*

Gram-negative rods
○ Enterobacteria (e.g. *E. coli, Shigella, Salmonella, Yersinia, Klebsiella, Proteus*)
○ Parvobacteria (*Brucella, Bordatella, Haemophilus*)
○ *Vibrio, Campylobacter, Pseudomonas, Legionella*
○ Anaerobes, e.g. *Bacteroides*

Other types of bacteria (Spirochaetales, Rickettsiaceae, Chlamydiae, Mycoplasma)

Gram-positive cocci

Staphylococci
- *Staph. aureus.*

CAUSES
- Localised infections: skin, otitis externa.
- Pneumonia (after influenza).
- Bacteraemia: may lead to endocarditis and bone or joint infections.
- Toxin-mediated disease: food poisoning, staphylococcal scalded skin syndrome, staphylococcal toxic shock syndrome.

TREATMENT   With a beta-lactam, e.g. flucloxacillin; vancomycin or teicoplanin if methicillin-resistant (MRSA).

Coagulase-negative staphylococci (e.g. Staph. epidermidis)
Causes infections associated with artificial joints (septic arthritis), valves (endocarditis), and other indwelling devices (e.g. CSF shunts).

TREATMENT   Usually with vancomycin or teicoplanin.

Streptococci
- **α-haemolytic:** *Strep. pneumoniae* (pneumococcus).
  Causes pneumonia, meningitis; viridans-type streptococci – endocarditis.
- **β-haemolytic:** *Strep. pyogenes* (group A).
  Causes soft tissue infections, pharyngitis, peritonsillar abscess (quinsy); toxin causes scarlet fever/toxic shock syndrome.
- **Group B:** *Strep. agalactiae.*
  Causes meningitis, pneumonia (in neonates).
- **Group D:** *Strep. bovis* and Enterococci (*E. faecalis* or *E. faecium*).
  Causes endocarditis, UTI, intra-abdominal infections, wound infections.
- Streptococcus 'milleri' (often group F) is a cause of brain and liver abscesses.

TREATMENT   Most streptococci are penicillin-sensitive although resistance is increasing. Endocarditis generally requires a penicillin and an aminoglycoside (*see Cardiology* section).

Gram-positive rods

Diphtheria – Corynebacterium diphtheriae
- Causes sore throat with a pharyngeal 'pseudomembrane', lymphadenopathy, 'bull neck' secondary to oedema. Occasionally systemic involvement secondary to toxin effects (particularly myocarditis and motor neuropathy).
- Treatment: acutely with antitoxin and antibiotics (e.g. erythromycin). Vaccination (as part of DTP vaccine) means it is rare in the UK. More common in Russia.

Listeriosis – Listeria monocytogenes
- Caused by eating raw or undercooked food, e.g. soft cheeses. Rare in healthy adults.
- Causes meningitis (or encephalitis), particularly in the elderly. If it occurs in pregnancy, it can lead to neonatal infection and premature labour.
- Treatment: with intravenous ampicillin and aminoglycoside (e.g. gentamicin).

Anthrax – Bacillus anthracis
- Extremely rare. Spread via contact with animals/animal products.
- Three forms of disease: *cutaneous* (ulcerating painless inflamed nodule that becomes a black scab, with surrounding oedema); *pulmonary* (pneumonia); and *GI* (abdominal pain and watery diarrhoea).
- Treatment: with ciprofloxacin. Vaccination is available to those at risk.

Gram-negative cocci
Neisseria
- *N. meningitidis* (meningococcus) – *see Neurology* section.
- *N. gonorrhoeae* (gonococcus) – *see Sexually Transmitted Diseases* below.

Gram-negative rods
Enterobacteriaceae
- *See Intestinal Infections* below.
- The most common cause of UTIs – in particular *E. coli, Proteus mirabilis, Klebsiella* sp.

Parvobacteria
- **Brucella:** *B. abortus, suis, melitensis* (brucellosis or undulant/Malta fever).
- **Bordetella:** *B. pertussis* (whooping cough).
- **Haemophilus:** *H. influenzae* (meningitis, pneumonia, skin, septic arthritis).

Other gram-negative rods
- **Vibrio** – *see Intestinal Infections* below.
- **Campylobacter** – *see Intestinal Infections* below.
- **Pseudomonas:** *Ps. aeruginosa* (pneumonia, UTI, skin), *Ps. mallei* (glanders).
- **Legionella:** *L. pneumophila* (pneumonia = Legionnaire's disease).

Spirochaetes
- **Treponema:** *T. pallidum* causes syphilis. Other treponemal diseases are bejel, yaws and pinta.
- **Leptospirosis:** from freshwater contaminated by animal (e.g. rat) urine. Most infections are subclinical but it can cause a febrile illness followed by a second phase with meningism, conjunctival haemorrhage and occasionally jaundice, tender hepatomegaly, haemorrhage and renal failure (Weil's disease).
- **Borreliosis:** Lyme disease (*Borrelia burgdorferi*) is spread by *Ixodes* ticks common in woodland areas where there are deer and sheep. Characteristic rash (erythema chronicum migrans) can be followed by a second phase with cardiac and neurological features, e.g. myocarditis, meningitis, cranial nerve palsies (e.g. seventh). Arthritis may occur late.

Rickettsiaceae
This group includes *Rickettsia, Coxiella* and *Bartonella*. Commonly carried by arthropod vectors such as lice, fleas, ticks and mites:
- **Rickettsiae** commonly cause typhus, a disease with swinging fever, headache and rash associated with vasculitis and multisystem involvement. Three groups: *typhus group* (epidemic and endemic typhus), *spotted fever group* (Rocky Mountain spotted fever, tick typhus, rickettsial pox) and *scrub typhus group*.
- **Coxiella** *burnetii* causes an atypical pneumonia (Q fever).
- **Bartonella** *henselae* causes cat scratch disease; *B. quintana* causes trench fever.

Chlamydiae
- Urethritis/Pelvic inflammatory disease (serovars D–K): *see STDs* below.
- Trachoma (serovars A–C): conjunctival infection and corneal scarring/ blindness.
- Lymphogranuloma venereum (LGV) (serovars L1–3): rare in developed world; causes painless genital ulceration then tender lymphadenopathy.

Mycoplasma
- *M. pneumoniae* causes an atypical pneumonia. Treatment: commonly sensitive to macrolides.

Anaerobic infections
Clostridium species
- *C. tetani* (tetanus): causes muscle spasms, e.g. 'lockjaw' (trismus).
- *C. botulinum* (botulism): causes a descending paralysis (initially cranial nerves with limb involvement later) and autonomic features (e.g. dilated pupils).
- *C. perfringens:* causes food poisoning and gas gangrene.
- *C. difficile* (pseudomembranous colitis): causes diarrhoea following antibiotic exposure.

Anaerobic sepsis
Organisms include *Bacteroides fragilis*, *Prevotella*, Fusobacteria.

9.2. Tuberculosis, leprosy and other mycobacterial infections
Tuberculosis (TB)
Caused by *Mycobacterium tuberculosis*, this is a common disease worldwide and a major public health concern, particularly with HIV co-infection. In the UK it is most prevalent among immigrants from the Indian subcontinent and Africa.

Primary TB: inhaled mycobacteria replicate in the lungs resulting in the formation of granulomas (Ghon foci). Hilar lymphadenopathy together with the granulomatous lesion is known as the primary complex. Although erythema nodosum may occur, primary TB is generally asymptomatic. The Ghon focus normally heals but with immunosuppression, reactivation may occur leading to:

Post-primary TB: reactivation of latent infection leads to pulmonary disease with classical symptoms of cough, haemoptysis, night sweats, fever, malaise and weight loss.

Extrapulmonary TB: in some cases post-primary TB presents with symptoms outside the lungs, e.g. meningitis, urogenital TB, TB of the spine (Pott's disease), and cervical lymphadenopathy (scrofula). Dissemination of TB throughout the body via the blood causes 'miliary TB' which may present non-specifically.

INVESTIGATIONS
- Sputum microscopy (acid-fast bacilli seen with Ziehl-Nielsen or auramine staining) and culture.
- Chest x-ray.
- Mantoux test may be positive.
- Non-respiratory tract samples – sometimes useful, e.g. early morning urine, ascitic tap for AFB.
- Occasionally, diagnosis is made from tissue biopsy showing (caseating) granulomas.

MANAGEMENT   Treatment of pulmonary TB is with four drugs (rifampicin and isoniazid for six months, with ethambutol and pyrazinamide for the first two months only). Pyridoxine is also given. There are cases, however, of multidrug-resistant TB. BCG vaccination offers protection against extrapulmonary (including CNS) TB.

Leprosy

Caused by *M. leprae* and occurs mostly in Asia. Clinical features depend on the immune response: a strong response causes tuberculoid leprosy; a weak response causes lepromatous leprosy; (borderline form in between).
- *Tuberculoid leprosy:* anaesthetic skin lesions with a hypopigmented centre; thickened nerves and neuropathies.
- *Lepromatous leprosy:* skin becomes thickened which may lead to a leonine facies appearance. Nerve damage leads to neuropathies. Repetitive trauma to anaesthetic digits can lead to damage and ultimately loss.

TREATMENT   Rifampicin and dapsone are used for tuberculoid leprosy with the addition of clofazimine for lepromatous leprosy.

Other mycobacterial infections
- *M. avium intracellulare* (MAI) can cause disseminated infection, e.g. in HIV patients.
- *M. marinum, M. ulcerans* cause skin infections ('fish-tank' granuloma/Buruli ulcer).
- *M. kansasi, M. malmoense, M. xenopi* can cause an indolent lung infection similar to TB.

9.3. Antibiotics
Inhibitors of cell wall synthesis
Beta lactams
i)   Penicillins
- Penicillinase-sensitive: benzylpenicillin, phenoxymethylpenicillin (penicillin V).
  › *Benzylpenicillin – used for strepto-, meningo- and gonococcal infections.*
- Penicillinase-resistant: flucloxacillin.
  › *Used for staphylococcal skin infections, endocarditis, osteomyelitis.*
- Broad-spectrum: amoxicillin, ampicillin, co-amoxiclav (amoxicillin with clavulanic acid = Augmentin).
  › *Used for simple respiratory infections and UTIs (note many resistant species now).*
- Anti-pseudomonal: ticarcillin (with clavulanic acid = Timentin), piperacillin (with tazobactam = Tazocin).
  › *Used to cover both Gram+ and Gram– organisms, i.e. nosomial, abdominal and pseudomonal infections.*

ii) Cephalosporins
- First generation: cefalexin.
  › *Used for urinary tract infections.*
- Second generation: cefuroxime.
- Third generation: ceftriaxone, cefotaxime.
  › *Broad-spectrum antibiotics with many uses including pneumonia, meningitis, septicaemia, biliary-tract infections.*

iii) Carbapenems (imipenem, meropenem) and monobactams (aztreonam)

Vancomycin and teicoplanin
Used to treat infections caused by MRSA and coagulase-negative staphylococci.

Inhibitors of protein synthesis
Tetracyclines (e.g. tetracycline, doxycycline)
Used for chlamydial infections, Lyme disease, mycoplasma infections.

Aminoglycosides (e.g. gentamicin, amikacin, tobramycin)
Used for treatment of serious infections (often in conjunction with another antibiotic).

Macrolides (e.g. erythromycin, clarithromycin, azithromycin)
Used for treatment of respiratory infections (*see* section on pneumonia)

Others: chloramphenicol, clindamycin and fusidic acid

Inhibitors of DNA synthesis or function
Sulphonamides

Trimethoprim
Used for 'lower' urinary tract infections.

Quinolones (e.g. ciprofloxacin, levofloxacin, moxifloxacin)
Multiple uses including UTIs, respiratory tract, GI and bone/joint infections.

Metronidazole
Used for anaerobic infections.

Newer antibiotics: linezolid and Synercid (quinupristin and dalfopristin).

Basic guide to antibiotic therapy

Pneumonia	
Community-acquired	Amoxicillin (or macrolide if penicillin-allergic) if uncomplicated, or cefuroxime and macrolide if severe
'Atypical'	Macrolide
Hospital-acquired	Broad-spectrum cephalosporin, e.g. cefotaxime or antipseudomonal penicillin
'Lower' UTI	Trimethoprim or nitrofurantoin or amoxicillin or oral cephalosporin
Endocarditis	Penicillin (flucloxacillin, benzylpenicillin or amoxicillin depending on organism) and gentamicin (*see Cardiology* section)
Meningitis	Empiric treatment with benzylpenicillin or cephalosporin, e.g. cefotaxime. For meningococcus either benzylpenicillin or cefotaxime can be used; for pneumococcus and *H. influenzae* use cefotaxime; for *Listeria* use amoxicillin and gentamicin
Infective diarrhoea	May not need any treatment; ciprofloxacin if severe
Septic arthritis	Flucloxacillin and fusidic acid (clindamycin if penicillin allergy)
Cellulitis	Benzylpenicillin and flucloxacillin (erythromycin if penicillin allergy)

- As part of the immunisation schedule: diphtheria, tetanus, pertussis (DTP), H. influenzae B, Meningococcus C, BCG.
- Other bacterial vaccines available include: Pneumococcus, Typhoid, Anthrax.

9.4. Pyrexia of unknown origin (PUO)

Most patients who present with a fever lasting for >1–2 weeks will usually have received a diagnosis for their illness. However, rarely it remains unexplained and is known as a fever or pyrexia of unknown origin (FUO or PUO). PUO can be grouped according to cause:
- infection (e.g. endocarditis, osteomyelitis, TB, HIV)
- inflammation (e.g. autoimmune disorders such as SLE, vasculitis)
- malignancy (particularly haematological malignancies)
- drug-induced (e.g. antibiotics)
- factitious (rare).

A detailed history is important (including travel, occupational, pets or other animal contact, hobbies). Examination also has to be detailed. Investigations are guided by the history and the examination but include serological blood tests, imaging and echocardiography.

9.5. Fever in the returned traveller

Although many infections in returned travellers will be short-lived, bacterial or viral infections and malaria must be excluded. In rare circumstances, haemorrhagic viral fevers should also be considered and tropical medicine specialist advice should be taken. A detailed history of exactly where the patient has travelled is important. If any doubt regarding an infectious disease, isolate immediately.

9.6. Bacteraemia

This describes the presence of organisms in the blood and can be caused by any organism. Clinical features: bacteraemia can lead to serious illness – so-called 'septic shock' with rigors, confusion, hypotension, tachycardia and warm peripheries.

The most common cause is Gram-negative bacteria but other causes include *Staph. aureus*, pneumococcus and meningococcus. Management: supportive treatment is important including fluid resuscitation and inotropic support if indicated. Antibiotic therapy should be guided by the results of blood cultures (*see* section on *Sepsis*).

9.7. Viral infections

DNA viruses
- Herpesvirus (*see* below)
- Hepadnavirus: hepatitis B
- Papovavirus: human papillomavirus (HPV), JC virus
- Poxvirus: smallpox, cowpox, orf, molluscum contagiosum
- Others: parvovirus, adenovirus

RNA viruses
- Picornavirus: enterovirus (polio, Coxsackie, echo), rhinovirus, hepatitis A
- Togavirus: rubella, flavivirus (hepatitis C, yellow fever, dengue fever)
- Calicivirus: Norwalk, hepatitis E
- Paramyxovirus: measles, mumps, parainfluenza, RSV
- Others: orthomyxovirus (influenza), rhabdovirus (rabies), reovirus (rotavirus)

Retroviruses – these are RNA viruses which are reverse transcribed into DNA
- ○ Human immunodeficiency virus (HIV)
- ○ Human T-cell lymphotropic virus (HTLV)

- Parvovirus B19 causes erythema infectiosum (fifth disease) in children with a facial rash ('slapped cheek' appearance). It can also precipitate an aplastic crisis in patients with chronic haemolysis, e.g. sickle cell disease.
- Enteroviruses can cause fever, URTI, GI upset, rash, meningo-encephalitis
  - ▸ *Polioviruses* very rarely can cause poliomyelitis (asymmetric flaccid paralysis affecting the lower limbs more than the upper with no sensory involvement).
  - ▸ *Coxsackie viruses* cause hand, foot and mouth disease, myocarditis, pleurodynia (Bornholm's disease) and herpangina.
- Rubella causes a prodromal illness with lymphadenopathy and Forchheimer spots; this is followed by a pinkish-red maculopapular rash. Congenital infection can produce a syndrome with cardiac, ocular and neurological problems.
- Mumps causes a prodrome followed by parotitis. Complications include meningitis, epididymo-orchitis and pancreatitis.
- Measles causes coryza, cough, conjunctivitis and Koplik's spots followed by a maculopapular rash which initially presents on the face and spreads over the rest of the body. Complications such as encephalitis are very rare.

Vaccination
- ○ As part of immunisation schedule: MMR (measles, mumps and rubella) and polio
- ○ Others available: influenza, hepatitis A and B, yellow fever, rabies, Japanese B encephalitis

Antivirals
- ○ *See* below for drugs used in herpes and HIV viruses
- ○ Other agents include:
  - ▸ ribavirin (RSV, hepatitis C)
  - ▸ amantadine (influenza A)
  - ▸ the neuraminidase inhibitors, e.g. zanamivir and oseltamivir (influenza)
  - ▸ the interferons (hepatitis B and C)

9.8. HIV

The human immunodeficiency virus (HIV) is a major worldwide cause of morbidity and mortality. HIV-1 and 2 are lentiviruses (part of the retrovirus family): HIV-1 is found worldwide but HIV-2 is found mainly in West Africa. HIV attacks CD4 cells causing immune dysfunction. Transmission is sexually, via blood, or via the mother to her foetus (either at birth or via breastfeeding).

Seroconversion: this can take up to three months, from initial infection to the presence of antibodies in the blood. Some patients will have a seroconversion illness during this period with fever, malaise, lymphadenopathy and rash. However, the majority of patients will be asymptomatic. Following seroconversion, patients may remain well for weeks to many years later. However, as CD4 levels decrease (and viral load increases) opportunistic infections and tumours begin to occur.

CLINICAL FEATURES
Respiratory
- *Pneumocystis jirovecii* (formally known as *Pneumocystis carinii*) is a fungus which causes pneumonia (pneumocystis pneumonia or PCP): dry cough,

dyspnoea and fever but with few signs on examination of the chest. Patients may be hypoxic, particularly after exercise. Diagnosis: can be made following staining of a bronchoalveolar lavage. Treatment: co-trimoxazole, clindamycin/primaquine or pentamidine. Steroids are given in severe illnesses when patients are hypoxic.
- TB is commonly seen in HIV-positive patients. Other mycobacterial infections seen include *Mycobacterium avium intracellulare (MAI)*.
- Other fungi that can affect the lung include *Aspergillus* and *Histoplasma*.

Neuro-ophthalmic
- *Cytomegalovirus* (CMV): retinitis, encephalitis.
- TB: subacute meningitis, focal neurological signs secondary to tuberculoma.
- *Toxoplasmosis* (*see Protozoa* below).
- *Cryptococcus:* meningitis.
- Progressive multifocal leucoencephalopathy (PML) is caused by JC virus.
- CNS lymphoma.
- HIV itself may cause retinitis, encephalopathy (dementia), myelopathy, neuropathy.

Gastrointestinal
- Candidiasis: can be oral or oesophageal.
- Oral hairy leucoplakia (associated with Epstein-Barr virus, EBV).
- Diarrhoea: can be caused by CMV, cryptosporidia and other fungi, as well as by infections that affect the immunocompetent (*see Gut Infections*). Note that diarrhoea can also be caused by tumours (Kaposi's sarcoma, lymphoma) and as a side effect of some antiretrovirals.

Skin
- Kaposi's sarcoma: caused by HHV8; this is a vascular tumour which causes purple nodular lesions on the skin or mucous membranes (and lungs/GI tract).

Note that patients with HIV also commonly suffer infections that immunocompetent patients contract and these should always be considered.

AIDS (Acquired immunodeficiency syndrome) is a term used to describe advanced HIV infection with the presence of certain opportunistic infections or tumours. However, with improved antiretroviral therapy and as these infections/tumours have become more treatable (at least in the developed world) this term has become less useful.

MANAGEMENT   Monitoring of CD4 T-cell count and HIV RNA level (viral load) is important. The CD4 T-cell count reflects the susceptibility to (opportunistic) infections; the viral load is inversely related to the rate of CD4 T-cell decline.

Treatment of HIV is with highly active antiretroviral therapy (HAART), which consists of a combination of three (or four) drugs from the following groups:
1. Reverse transcriptase inhibitors (RTIs).
   - *Nucleoside RTIs:* zidovudine (AZT), lamivudine (3TC), didanosine (ddI), zalcitabine (ddC), abacavir, emtricitabine (FTC).
   - *Nucleotide RTIs:* tenofovir.
   - *Non-Nucleoside RTIs:* efavirenz, nevirapine.

2. Protease inhibitors (PIs).
   - (fos)amprenavir, atazanavir, darunavir, nelfinavir, indinavir, saquinavir, lopinavir and ritonavir, a PI that in low dose inhibits CYP3A4-mediated

elimination of co-administered PIs, resulting in more favourable ('boosted') plasma concentrations of these PIs.

3. Entry inhibitors.
    » *Fusion inhibitors:* enfurvitide.
    » *CCR5 inhibitors:* miraviroc.

Common combinations include: two NRTIs + one NNRTI, or two NRTIs + one boosted PI.

Indications for HAART treatment: if symptomatic, and in asymptomatic patients if CD4 count drops between 200 and 350; hence the importance of close monitoring of CD4 count.

Side effect of HAART therapy

Many of the HAART drugs can cause nausea, diarrhoea and rashes. Specific side effects of some of the drugs include:
○ AZT – bone marrow suppression, anaemia
○ ddI/ddC – peripheral neuropathy, pancreatitis
○ Efavirenz – vivid dreams, depression

9.9. Hepatitis viruses

Some viruses commonly cause acute hepatitis and others chronic hepatitis:
● **Acute hepatitis:** clinical features: non-specific malaise with nausea, vomiting, fever, abdominal pain and jaundice.
● **Chronic hepatitis:** chronic infection with a hepatitis virus may be asymptomatic, or result in chronic hepatitis which may progress to cirrhosis with features of chronic liver disease and hepatocellular carcinoma.

Hepatitis A
RNA virus (picornavirus) with faeco-oral transmission. Clinical features: causes an acute illness with no chronic form. Anti-HAV IgM antibodies will be present. Treatment is supportive and a vaccine is available.

Hepatitis B
DNA virus (hepadnavirus) with blood-borne, sexual or materno-foetal transmission. Clinical features: causes an acute illness (often mild), after which ≈ 5–10% of patients will become chronic carriers. Complications: vasculitis, glomerulonephritis and arthropathy. Investigations: acute infection is characterised by the presence of anti-HBc IgM (antibodies to core antigen) and chronic infection by HBsAg (surface antigen). The presence of HBeAg (e antigen) denotes a high rate of viral replication and infectiousness. If infection is cleared, antibodies to these antigens become detectable. Treatment of acute hepatitis B is supportive; chronic disease may be treated with alpha-interferon, lamivudine, adefovir, entecavir, tenofovir and emtricitane. A vaccine is available.

Hepatitis C
RNA virus (flavivirus) with blood-borne or sexual transmission (former more common). Acute infection is generally mild but leads to chronic carriage in 60–80% of patients. Complications: cryoglobulinaemia. Treatment of chronic hepatitis C infection includes alpha interferon and ribavirin. There is currently no vaccine.

Hepatitis D

This is a defective RNA virus that requires co-infection with hepatitis B virus in order to replicate in the human body. It can worsen hepatitis B.

Hepatitis E

RNA virus (calicivirus) with faeco-oral transmission. Clinical features: causes acute hepatitis without chronic illness. Anti-HEV IgM is diagnostic. Treatment is supportive. Mortality is high in pregnancy.

Herpes viruses (*see* below) and yellow fever viruses may also cause acute hepatitis.

9.10. Herpes infections

Herpes viruses are DNA viruses. They can be divided into three families (α, β, γ) and are able to persist in a latent state in an infected organism with periodic reactivation.

Alphaherpesvirus

Herpes simplex virus (HSV-1 and 2)

- Spread by direct/sexual contact.
- Clinical features: ulcers (HSV-1 commonly oropharyngeal mucosa, HSV-2 genitals and anus); may also cause keratitis, encephalitis and rarely a disseminated infection.

Varicella zoster virus (VZV)

Causes chicken pox (varicella) and shingles (zoster). The majority of adults are seropositive.

- Varicella occurs mainly in children – rarely recurrent. Often there is a non-specific prodromal illness followed by fever and an itchy rash over the face, scalp and trunk that progresses from macules through to papules and vesicles to pustules. Complications include secondary bacterial or disseminated infection.
- Zoster causes similar skin lesions to varicella but is commonly unilateral and limited to a dermatomal distribution (normally the trunk but can affect the face) with pain in that area (that can occur before the rash). Complications include post-herpetic neuralgia (particularly in older patients) and Ramsay Hunt syndrome.

Betaherpesvirus

Cytomegalovirus (CMV)

Often asymptomatic but can cause an infectious mononucleosis-like illness. Complications such as encephalitis, retinitis, pancytopenia, colitis and adrenal disease are more common in the immunocompromised (HIV or transplant patients).

Human herpes virus (HHV-6 and HHV-7)

These viruses can cause a childhood illness with fever/rash (exanthem subitum).

Gammaherpesvirus

Epstein-Barr virus (EBV)

Causes infectious mononucleosis ('glandular fever'). Primary infection (after an incubation period of around one month) causes fever, sore throat, headache, malaise and cervical lymphadenopathy. Less common features are splenomegaly, hepatomegaly and jaundice. Investigations: blood tests show a lymphocytosis with 'atypical lymphocytes'; 'Monospot' test is positive. EBV is also associated with lymphoma and nasopharyngeal carcinoma.

Human herpes virus (HHV-8)

Associated with Kaposi's sarcoma, a vascular tumour commonly affecting the skin, and Castleman's disease.

Antivirals used in the treatment of herpes viruses

○ Aciclovir (valaciclovir, famciclovir) – used for HZV/VZV, it is a chain terminator of viral DNA synthesis after phosphorylation of α and γ virus-encoded thymidine kinase
○ Ganciclovir (valganciclovir), cidofovir and foscarnet – used for CMV

9.11. Fungi

Yeasts

Candida (albicans most common)

- In immunocompetent individuals, causes a local infection (e.g. vaginal or oral thrush, nappy rash, paronychia); treat topically, e.g. clotrimazole or nystatin.
- In immunocompromised individuals, other infections are seen (e.g. oesophagitis) requiring systemic treatment, e.g. fluconazole.

Cryptococcus neoformans

Spread by birds and enters via respiratory tract. Most common presentation is subacute meningitis. Rarely, dissemination with cryptococcoma in liver, spleen or other viscera. Investigations: India ink stain of CSF or cryptococcal antigen in serum/CSF. Treatment is with intravenous amphotericin +/– flucytosine, followed by fluconazole.

Moulds or filamentous fungi

Aspergillus (e.g. fumigatus)

3 major forms of the disease.

- Allergic bronchopulmonary aspergillosis (ABPA).
- Aspergilloma.
- Invasive aspergillosis: may lead to pneumonia or meningitis.

Dermatophytes

These are a group of fungi causing chronic fungal infections of skin, hair and nails. Often known as tinea or 'ringworm', they have characteristic fluorescence under Wood's (UV) light.

- Tinea corporis: itchy, red rash with a raised edge and a lighter centre, over the limbs and trunk.
- Tinea pedis ('athlete's foot').
- Tinea capitis (scalp).
- Tinea cruris (groin).

MANAGEMENT   Topical treatment with an azole except for nail or scalp involvement when systemic therapy is required (e.g. terbinafine, itraconazole).

Dimorphic species (yeast in the host but moulds in vitro)
Histoplasmosis (e.g. capsulatum)
CLINICAL FEATURES   Inhaled spores lead to pulmonary involvement. Chronic disease may be difficult to distinguish from TB.

Anti-fungals (important side effects within brackets)
- Polyenes: e.g. amphotericin (*nephrotoxicity*), nystatin.
- Azoles: topical, e.g. clotrimazole; or systemic, e.g. ketoconazole, fluconazole, itraconazole, voriconazole, posaconazole (*hepatoxicity*).
- Allylamines: e.g. terbinafine.
- Echinocandins: e.g. caspofungin.
- Others include flucytosine (*bone marrow suppression*).

9.12. Protozoa

Important protozoal infections
- ○ *Toxoplasma* (*see* below)
- ○ *Trichomonas vaginalis:* causes urethritis with frothy grey/green discharge
- ○ *Giardia lamblia* and *Entamoeba histolytica* (*see Intestinal Infections*)
- ○ *Cryptosporidium*
- ○ *Plasmodium* (*see Malaria*)
- ○ *Trypanosoma* (*see Other tropical infections* – Trypanosomiasis)
- ○ *Leishmania* (*see Other tropical infections* – Leishmaniasis)

Toxoplasmosis – toxoplasma gondii
- Spread: oocysts in cat faeces, tissue cysts in undercooked meat or transplacentally.
- Commonly asymptomatic although may cause an infectious mononucleosis-type illness acutely. Seropositivity is variable in different areas.
- Infection becomes latent, with the immunocompromised most at risk of reactivation. Common clinical features – *Ocular:* uveitis or chorioretinitis; *Cerebral:* focal neurological signs with seizures, headaches, altered consciousness, fever; ring-enhancing lesions seen on brain imaging.
- Treatment is with pyrimethamine and sulphadiazine; spiramycin in pregnancy.

9.13. Helminths

Important helminthic infections
Nematodes (roundworms)
- ○ Filaria (*see Other tropical infections* – Filariasis)
- ○ Gut (*see Intestinal Infections*)
- ○ *Toxocara* (*see* below)

Cestodes (tapeworms)
- ○ *Taenia* (*see* below)
- ○ *Echinococcus* cause hydatid disease with liver or lung cysts the most common feature

Trematodes (flukes)
- ○ *Schistosoma* (*see Other tropical infections* – Schistosomiasis)

Toxocara canis (dogs) or cati (cats)
Spread by faeces or infected food. Causes *larva migrans:* visceral (migration to liver

and lungs with fever, wheeze, lymphadenopathy and hepatosplenomegaly) or ocular (migration to eye with pain and decreased acuity).

Taenia saginata (beef) or solium (pork)
Can grow many metres within the upper jejunum. Majority are asymptomatic or cause mild abdominal pain. Cysticercosis occurs when the larval stage of *T. solium* invades tissues and becomes encysted: there are three forms – cerebral (space-occupying lesions with focal neurological signs and seizures), ocular and subcutaneous (hard nodules).

9.14. Malaria
This is a disease of hot, humid countries in areas <2000 m above sea level. It is caused by a species of the protozoa *Plasmodium* (*falciparum* and the three 'benign' malarias *vivax*, *ovale* and *malariae*), and is spread by the female *Anopheles* mosquito.
   There are three stages in the life-cycle of plasmodia species:
- **Pre-erythrocytic stage:** the mosquito injects *sporozoites* into the human circulation. They pass to the liver where they form tissue *schizonts*. These rupture and release *merozoites* which re-enter the bloodstream and invade red blood cells.
- **Erythrocytic stage:** the merozoites continue multiplying within the red blood cells and when the cells rupture many merozoites are released, infecting new cells and causing fever.
- **Exo-erythrocytic stage:** not all schizonts in the liver rupture – in *vivax* and *ovale* the merozoites produce *hypnozoites*, which lie dormant in the liver for months/years leading to late relapses.

CLINICAL FEATURES
- Non-specific prodrome followed by rigors and fever which are classically periodic: every 48 hours (or 72 hours in *P. malariae*). Three stages are described: 'cold', 'hot', 'sweating'.
- *P. vivax* and *P. ovale* infections are generally not severe but can cause relapse. *P. malariae* is also normally mild but can be chronic and lead to nephrotic syndrome.
- *P. falciparum* infection is usually more severe and can affect most organs of the body, rapidly leading to multi-organ failure and death.
  - Cerebral malaria (encephalopathy with decreased consciousness and seizures).
  - Anaemia (secondary to haemolysis).
  - Renal failure.
  - Pulmonary oedema.
  - Hepatitis/jaundice and hepatosplenomegaly.

INVESTIGATIONS
- Microscopy of thick and thin blood films.
- Antigen detection tests are also available.

MANAGEMENT
- Supportive measures are important in falciparum malaria.
- Antimalarial drugs include:
  - non-falciparum: chloroquine; for vivax/ovale this should be followed by a course of primaquine to eliminate risk of relapse
  - falciparum: quinine PO or IV if severe, followed by Fansidar. Side effects of quinine include hypoglycaemia (monitor closely with IV), nausea and tinnitus

- Prophylaxis: avoid being bitten (mosquito nets, repellents and covering body); drugs depending on area visited (mefloquine, Malarone, doxycyline).

9.15. Other tropical infections
Leishmaniasis
Various protozoal species spread by sandflies of genus *Phlebotomus* in (sub)tropical areas of Africa and Asia, and *Lutzomyia* in South America.

Visceral leishmaniasis – Kala-azar
Mainly caused by *L. donovani*. Clinical features: fever, dry and rough skin which may become pigmented, and massive hepatosplenomegaly.

Cutaneous leishmaniasis
Caused by various Leishmania species. Clincal features: single or multiple painless nodules over the face or extremities at the site of the bite. These may ulcerate with a red raised border and heal very slowly leaving a scar. A mucocutaneous type in South America is known as espundia.

Trypanosomiasis
African trypanosomiasis – sleeping sickness
Protozoa spread by tsetse fly (*Glossina* sp.). Two main types: *T. brucei gambiense* (West Africa) and *T. brucei rhodesiense* (East Africa). Clinical features: the bite causes a chancre (tender nodule) followed by multiorgan involvement.
- Lymphadenopathy and hepatosplenomegaly.
- Chronic meningoencephalitis (behavioural changes, apathy, falling asleep).
- Myocarditis.

South American trypanosomiasis – Chagas' disease
T. cruzi is spread by Reduviid insects. Three phases.
- Acute: chagoma (papule at site of bite), hepatosplenomegaly, fever, rash.
- Latent period which may last years.
- Chronic: affecting heart (cardiomyopathy) and GI (achalasia, megacolon).

Schistosomiasis – bilharzia
A fluke infection with the snail as a vector which has several stages:
- Free swimming larval cercariae penetrate the skin causing a local itchy lesion.
- Following this there is a generalised allergic response with fever, urticaria and enlarged lymph nodes.
- Lastly, after egg production urinary or bowel symptoms predominate depending on where the organism migrates. *S. haematobium* causes haematuria and may lead to chronic urinary symptoms and renal failure. *S. japonicum* and *S. mansoni* cause bloody diarrhoea.

Treatment is with praziquantel.

Filariasis
Lymphatic filaria (*Brugia malayi, Wuchereria bancrofti*) are spread via mosquitoes and cause episodic fever and lymphangitis. Recurrent infections may cause fibrosis of the lymphatics (elephantiasis). Skin filaria include *Onchocerca volvulus* which is transmitted by the black fly and invades the skin and eyes (River blindness).

9.16. Sexually transmitted diseases

STDs in men

Urethritis

Causes urethral discharge and dysuria although rarely can be asymptomatic. Local complications may occur, e.g. prostatitis and epididymitis.

- Gonococcal urethritis (gonorrhoea): caused by *Neisseria gonorrhoeae* (gonococcus). Rarely systemic infection affecting skin (petechiae, pustules) and joint (tenosynovitis, arthritis) is seen. Treatment: antibiotic therapy depends on local sensitivities but usually treatment is with a third generation cephalosporin (e.g. cefuroxime).
- Non-gonococcal urethritis: caused by *Chlamydia trachomatis* and other organisms such as *Mycoplasma genitalium* and *Ureaplasma urealyticum*. Treatment: recommended regimens are single dose azithromycin or seven days of doxycycline.

STDs in women

As with men, infections can be split into gonococcal and non-gonococcal. *Chlamydia* is the most common cause. Frequently asymptomatic but pelvic inflammatory disease (PID) can develop with variable symptoms including lower abdominal pain, dysuria, vaginal discharge. Extrapelvic complications include perihepatitis (Fitz-Hugh-Curtis syndrome). Chronically, PID can result in infertility, chronic pelvic pain and is a risk factor for ectopic pregnancy.

Bacterial vaginosis

Vaginal discharge with a fishy smell. No evidence that it is a sexually transmitted disease. Aetiology: alteration of the bacterial flora in the vagina with increase in species such as *Gardnerella vaginalis* and anaerobes. Clue cells are seen. Treatment: antibiotics such as metronidazole.

Genital ulcers

Can be painful or painless.

- *Painful: Herpes simplex* (most common), chancroid and rarely Behcet's disease or ulcerative skin disorders such as pemphigus.
- *Painless:* syphilis, granuloma inguinale, LGV, squamous cell carcinoma.

Genital warts

Common – caused by human papillomaviruses (HPV). Usually multiple and can occur anywhere around the genital area. Treatment: options include topical podophyllotoxin, imiquimod or cryotherapy.

Syphilis

Acquired syphilis is classified as either early, i.e. within two years of infection (primary, secondary and early latent, i.e. asymptomatic) and late (tertiary and late latent).

- ○ EARLY: Primary causes a painless ulcer known as a chancre; secondary causes multisystem involvement within first two years with symmetrical pustular rash on palms/soles, 'snail-track' ulcers, condylomata lata, lymphadenopathy
- ○ LATE: most commonly late latent (i.e. asymptomatic) but can be (1) gummas in skin, bone and rarely viscera; (2) cardiovascular (e.g. aortitis) or (3) neurological (general paresis, tabes dorsalis, meningovascular)

Management: first line treatment is with IM procaine penicillin, duration depends on the type.

9.17. Intestinal infections

Diarrhoea may be watery through to bloody (dysentery). Vomiting, abdominal pain and fever are also seen. Management: first-line treatment is oral rehydration therapy. Antibiotics are rarely needed – ciprofloxacin is first choice if bacterial cause suspected.

Viruses
- *Rotavirus:* mainly young children.
- *Calicivirus* (Norwalk or SRSV): causes winter vomiting disease.
- CMV: in the immunosuppressed.

Bacterial
- *Campylobacter jejuni:* commonest cause of infective diarrhoea in the UK.
- *Escherichia coli:* ETEC (enterotoxigenic) and EPEC (enteropathogenic) cause watery diarrhoea; EIEC (enteroinvasive) and EHEC (enterohaemorrhagic, including 0157) produces a more severe dysenteric illness. Haemolytic uraemic syndrome (HUS) may occur following EHEC infection.
- Salmonellae: causes enteric fever (typhoid caused by *S. typhi* or paratyphoid caused by *S. paratyphi*), or food poisoning (*S. enteritidis*). Rarely it produces a localised infection (e.g. osteomyelitis – particularly in sickle cell disease).
- Shigellae: *S. sonnei* causes mild infections; *S. dysenteriae, S. flexneri* and *S. boydii* cause dysentery.
- *Vibrio cholerae:* causes diarrhoea with 'rice water' stools leads to severe dehydration.

Protozoa
- Amoebiasis (*Entamoeba histolytica*): often insidious onset with few or mild symptoms but may lead to a fulminant colitis. Complications: toxic megacolon, amoeboma in colon and liver abscess. Treatment: with metronidazole +/– diloxanide furoate.
- *Giardia lamblia*: causes a watery diarrhoea with bloating and offensive flatus.
- *Cryptosporidium parvum, Isospora belli* and Microsporidiae: produces profound watery diarrhoea in the immunosuppressed, particularly HIV.

Helminths
- *Strongyloides stercoralis*: there may be accompanying skin signs (larva currens) and upper airway irritation.
- *Trichuris trichiuria* (whipworm): may cause rectal prolapse.
- *Enterobius vermicularis* (threadworm): causes pruritus ani.
- *Ascaris lumbricoides* (roundworm): may lead to bowel obstruction.
- *Ancylostoma duodenale* (hookworm): causes anaemia.

Toxin-mediated food poisoning
Causes include *Bacillus cereus* (often from rice), *Staphylococcus aureus, Clostridium perfringens, Vibrio parahaemolyticus* (from shellfish).

10

Haematology

10.1. LEUKAEMIAS

The leukaemias are defined as acute or chronic.
- Acute lymphoblastic (ALL).
- Acute myeloid (AML).
- Chronic lymphocytic (CLL).
- Chronic myeloid (CML).

Note that acute can be further subdivided, e.g. according to cytogenetics or cytological appearance (WHO classification). ALL is more common in children; AML and chronic leukaemias are more common in adults.

Possible aetiological factors: exposure to radiation or chemicals, e.g. benzene, previous cytotoxic chemotherapy. Proto-oncogenes can develop oncogenic potential through either mutations, e.g. Flt3 in AML, or chromosomal translocations, e.g. t(9:22) (the Philadelphia chromosome) in CML.

CLINICAL FEATURES There are common features that can occur in all of the leukaemias:
- Night sweats, weight loss, lymphadenopathy and hepatosplenomegaly.
- Pancytopenia-anaemia, neutropenia, thrombocytopenia.
- Infiltration of other tissues.

DIAGNOSIS Made from peripheral blood and bone marrow aspirate and trephine using morphological, immunophenotypic and cytogenetic techniques.

MANAGEMENT
- Acute: may involve chemotherapeutic agents and bone marrow transplantation in select patients.
- CML: imatinib mesylate, a tyrosine kinase inhibitor; other agents include alpha-interferon, busulphan or hydroxyurea; bone marrow transplantation may be considered.
- CLL: treatment is only indicated in certain situations (e.g. rapidly increasing lymphadenopathy or lymphocytosis). Chemotherapeutic agents can be used; radiotherapy may be helpful for bulky disease; bone marrow transplantation may be considered for younger patients.

Complications of treatment include: neutropenic sepsis and tumour lysis syndrome.

10.2. Lymphomas
Malignancies of lymphoid tissue.

Hodgkin's disease (HD)
Classified by histology and immunophenotypic markers as either:
- Nodular lymphocyte predominant (NLPHD) – best prognosis.
- Classical, which is further subdivided into:
  - nodular sclerosing
  - mixed cellularity
  - lymphocyte-deplete
  - lymphocyte-rich.

CLINICAL FEATURES   Patient may complain of 'B' symptoms (fever, night sweats, weight loss), and/or enlarged lymph nodes (particularly neck and mediastinum). Associated with Epstein-Barr virus.

DIAGNOSIS   From nodal biopsy – characteristic Reed-Sternberg cells.

INVESTIGATIONS
- Staging from CT imaging.
- Bone marrow biopsy.
- Blood tests – specifically FBC, LDH, LFTs, albumin, ESR.

TREATMENT   According to stage (Ann Arbor staging) and histological type:
- Localised NLPHD with radiotherapy only.
- Localised classical HD with chemotherapy and radiotherapy.
- Advanced disease with chemotherapy alone.

Non-Hodgkin's lymphoma
Classified into either B or T cell neoplasms. B cell tumours can be further subdivided into low-grade or high-grade tumours.

CLINICAL FEATURES   Wide clinical presentation including lymphadenopathy, 'B' symptoms, bone marrow suppression, hyperviscosity, hepatosplenomegaly, extranodal disease, e.g. skin rash. Associated with viruses, e.g. HTLV1, EBV, HIV, autoimmune disease, post-allogeneic organ transplant, exposure to radiation.

DIAGNOSIS   By lymph node/tissue biopsy.

MANAGEMENT
- Staging by bone marrow biopsy and CT scanning.
- Treatment is tailored to the type of tumour, i.e. B or T cell, high or low grade and the stage of tumour, and includes:
  - chemotherapy and/or radiotherapy
  - monoclonal antibodies, e.g. rituximab or alemtuzimab
  - bone marrow transplantation in select patients.

10.3. Myeloproliferative disorders
Chronic myeloid leukaemia
See above

Polycythaemia rubra vera
Primary proliferation of red cells within the bone marrow. Rarely there is transformation to acute leukaemia.

CLINICAL FEATURES
- Raised Hb and PCV.
- Splenomegaly.
- Pruritus.
- Increased risk of arterial and venous thrombosis.

MANAGEMENT
- Investigations: FBC, red cell mass (RCM), erythropoietin. Patients usually have a mutation in Jak2.
- Treatment: venesection and cytoreductives.

Essential thrombocythaemia
Primary proliferation of megakaryocytes leading to raised platelet count. Can transform to acute leukaemia or myelofibrosis.

CLINICAL FEATURES
- Arterial and venous thrombosis.
- Increased risk of bleeding due to platelet dysfunction.
- Splenomegaly.

MANAGEMENT
- Investigations: FBC, bone marrow aspirate and trephine, ferritin and CRP (to exclude secondary causes). Patients frequently have a mutation in Jak2.
- Treatment: aspirin, with the addition of cytoreductives in selected patients.

Idiopathic myelofibrosis
Primary proliferation of any or all myeloid cell lines, with associated bone marrow fibrosis. Can transform to acute leukaemia. Clinical features: massive splenomegaly and constitutional symptoms. Treatment is generally supportive, cytoreductives and bone marrow transplantation in selected patients.

10.4. Myelodysplastic syndrome
A spectrum of disorders where dysplastic features are seen in one or more myeloid cell line in the peripheral blood and bone marrow.

Incidence increases with age. Anaemia is the most common feature but pancytopenia may occur. Commonly transforms to acute myeloid leukaemia (AML).

Treatment is supportive with packed red blood cell and platelet transfusions, and antibiotics for neutropenic sepsis. Intensive chemotherapy and bone marrow transplantation can be used in a small percentage of patients.

10.5. Myeloma

Plasma cell tumour that secretes monoclonal immunoglobulin (paraprotein) or light chains. Paraproteins and light chains can be detected in the blood. Light chains may also be seen as Bence-Jones protein (BJP) in the urine.

There are many ways in which patients can present, e.g. bone pain, fractures, anaemia, renal failure, hypercalcaemia.

Diagnosis is based on detecting serum paraprotein, serum free light chains, or urinary BJP and increased plasma cells in bone marrow (>10%), in association with evidence of end-organ damage, i.e. anaemia, hypercalcaemia, renal failure, peripheral neuropathy, lytic lesions on plain x-ray or MRI, amyloid.

Renal failure is multifactorial: NSAIDs (taken for bone pain), hypercalcaemia causing calcium deposition, proximal tubular damage secondary to light-chain deposition, amyloid.

Treatment may involve chemotherapy. Other management is supportive and includes bisphosphonates to control hypercalcaemia, analgesia and radiotherapy for bone pain.

Worse prognosis with amyloid, raised Beta2 microglobulin, low albumin.

Monoclonal gammopathy of unknown significance (MGUS) is differentiated from myeloma by low paraprotein levels (<30 g/l), low plasma cell infiltration in bone marrow (<10%), and no evidence of end-organ damage.

10.6. Amyloid

This occurs when there is deposition of amyloid protein in tissues, including heart, peripheral nerves, kidneys, liver and tongue.

AL amyloid is composed of monoclonal light chains and is often found in association with myeloma.

AA amyloid is found in association with chronic inflammatory processes, e.g. rheumatoid arthritis.

Diagnosis is made when tissue biopsy demonstrates apple green birefringence under polarised light following staining with Congo red, and using Serum Amyloid P (SAP) scanning in specialist centres. Treatment of AL amyloid is similar to that for symptomatic myeloma; treatment of AA amyloid requires management of the chronic inflammatory state.

10.7. Bleeding disorders

Bleeding tendencies may be due to abnormalities of:
- Platelets.
- Clotting factors (coagulation).
- The vascular wall.

Bleeding disorders – platelets

Bleeding due to low platelet count or abnormal function of platelets.

CLINICAL FEATURES   Bleeding usually occurs in skin (purpura, bruising), gums, nose and other mucosal surfaces.

INVESTIGATIONS Platelet function can be measured using platelet aggregation studies to various *in vitro* agonists (bleeding time now rarely used). These assays are usually prolonged when platelet count falls below 100×10^9/l or in presence of qualitative defect.

Causes of thrombocytopenia

Failure of platelet production
○ Hereditary thrombocythaemia
○ Vitamin B12/folate deficiency
○ Marrow infiltration: e.g. carcinoma, lymphoma
○ Marrow suppressors: e.g. alcohol, viruses
○ Paroxysmal nocturnal haemoglobinuria

Increased platelet destruction
Immune causes
○ Idiopathic autoimmune thrombocytopenic purpura (ITP)
○ Secondary autoimmune thrombocytopenic purpura: e.g. SLE
○ Drugs: e.g. heparin
○ Post-transfusion

Nonimmune causes
○ Disseminated Intravascular Coagulation (DIC)
○ Haemolytic Uraemic Syndrome (HUS)/Thrombotic Thrombocytopenic Purpura (TTP)

Pooling in an enlarged spleen

Idiopathic autoimmune thrombocytopenic purpura (ITP)
Autoimmune disorder. Acute (more common in children) or chronic (more common in adults).

CLINICAL FEATURES
● Petechiae, ecchymoses, nose/gum bleeding.
● Acute form often preceded by viral infection.

DIAGNOSIS Is one of exclusion based on a normal FBC and blood film except for thrombocytopenia.

MANAGEMENT
● Acute ITP usually remits spontaneously.
● Corticosteroids or intravenous immunoglobulins can increase the platelet count in cases of severe bleeding.
● Chronic ITP may respond to corticosteroids or immunoglobulins but often relapses in up to 80% of cases.
● Second-line therapies include splenectomy, monoclonal antibodies (e.g. rituximab), and immunosuppression.

10.8. Bleeding disorders – clotting factors
● Clotting cascade consists of intrinsic, extrinsic, and common pathways.
● Disorders of intrinsic and common pathways identified by prolonged APTT.
● Disorders of extrinsic and common pathways identified by prolonged PT.
● Disorders of fibrinogen identified by prolonged thrombin time (TT).

Inherited disorders of coagulation
Haemophilia A
X-linked, affecting males, due to factor VIII deficiency which can be mild (>5% VIII level), moderate (1–5%) or severe (<1%). Clinical features: bleeding into deep tissues such as muscles and joints. Diagnosis: based on a normal PT but prolonged APTT which corrects with the addition of normal plasma. Treatment: intravenous recombinant factor VIII concentrate, either prophylactically (in severe disease) or at the earliest opportunity after bleeding commences. DDAVP can be given for mild or moderate cases.

Haemophilia B (Christmas disease)
X-linked, due to factor IX deficiency with mild, moderate and severe forms. Diagnosis: APTT prolonged, PT normal. Treatment: intravenous recombinant factor IX either prophylactically or to cessate bleeding. DDAVP is not effective.

Von Willebrand's disease
Autosomal disease due to abnormality or deficiency in Von Willebrand factor (VWF). VWF has two roles: first, to bind to the endothelial surface and platelets; second, to act as a carrier for factor VIII. Patients suffer from ecchymoses and nose bleeds. Diagnosis: based on a prolonged APTT, reduced factor VIII, reduced levels of VWF antigen and impaired ristocetin-induced platelet aggregation. Treatment: with tranexamic acid, DDAVP or VWF concentrate.

Acquired disorders of coagulation
Disseminated intravascular coagulation
Generalised activation of the clotting cascade followed by activation of the fibrinolytic pathway. Causes: sepsis, cancer and obstetric emergencies, e.g. placental abruption, amniotic fluid embolus. Usually complicated by bleeding but may also cause microthrombi. Diagnosis: based on identification of thrombocytopenia, high APTT and PT, low fibrinogen concentration and raised fibrin degradation products. Management: requires treatment of the precipitating cause and supportive care with blood products if bleeding occurs.

Liver disease
Can cause a bleeding disorder due to reduced production of clotting factors, increased fibrinolysis and thrombocytopenia. Investigations: prolonged PT and APTT, and low fibrinogen.

10.9. Bleeding disorders – other
Anticoagulant drugs
- **Heparin** potentiates the action of antithrombin and in turn inhibits other coagulation factors. Unfractionated heparin prolongs the APTT and requires monitoring; low molecular weight heparin has only a minimal effect on the APTT and is usually not monitored. Complications: bleeding, heparin-induced thrombocytopenia (HIT), osteoporosis, alopecia.
- **Warfarin** can be given orally, unlike heparin, and is a vitamin K antagonist, therefore inhibits factors II, VII, IX and X. It prolongs the PT and requires monitoring via the international normalised ratio (INR).

Thrombophilia
Acquired risk factors for venous thrombosis
- Immobility.

- Surgery.
- Cancer.
- Pregnancy.
- Oestrogen containing contraception and hormone replacement.
- Nephrotic syndrome.
- Antiphospholipid syndrome: acquired thrombophilia, can present with thrombocytopenia, arterial and venous thrombosis and recurrent miscarriages, due to the presence of antiphospholipid antibodies (e.g. lupus anticoagulant, anti-cardiolipin antibodies). APTT prolonged as a result of antibodies interfering with the phospholipids used in the APTT assay. Associated with SLE and other autoimmune diseases. Treatment may be required with anti-platelet drugs and anticoagulation.

Inherited risk factors for venous thrombosis
- Antithrombin deficiency.
- Protein C deficiency.
- Protein S deficiency.
- Factor V Leiden mutation.

10.10 Red cell disorders
The anaemias
Anaemia
A haemoglobin (Hb) below the normal range. Normal range typically, for men is 13.5–17.5 g/dl and for women is 11.5–15.5 g/dl.

CAUSES
- Reduced production of red blood cells.
- Increased loss or destruction of red cells.
- Increased plasma volume (dilutional).

CLINICAL FEATURES
- Tiredness.
- Lethargy.
- Shortness of breath.
- Chest pain if in association with ischemic heart disease.
- Heart failure (due to increased work load).
- Pallor.

Iron Deficiency Anaemia

Causes of iron deficiency anaemia
- ○ Bleeding: e.g. menorrhagia, gastrointestinal bleed
- ○ Reduced absorption of iron from the gut: e.g. coeliac disease
- ○ Poor diet (rare)

CLINICAL FEATURES
- Symptoms of anaemia (*see* above).
- Specific symptoms and signs: koilonychia, dysphagia due to oesophageal webs, atrophic glossitis.

DIAGNOSIS   Hypochromic, microcytic blood film, low serum ferritin and iron, high transferrin and low transferrin saturation.

TREATMENT   Requires establishment of the cause (e.g. OGD and colonoscopy) and replacing iron either orally, or intravenously if not tolerated orally.

Differential diagnosis for microcytosis

- ○ Iron deficiency anaemia
- ○ Thalassaemia
- ○ Sideroblastic anaemia (congenital and acquired, e.g. lead)
- ○ Anaemia of chronic disease (microcytosis mild)
- ○ Aluminium toxicity

Anaemia of chronic disease

Generally normochromic normocytic and develops secondary to a chronic underlying condition. Thought to be due to abnormal iron mobilisation into erythropoietic precursors. Diagnosis: based on normal/high ferritin, reduced iron and transferrin, reduced total iron binding capacity (TIBC).

Macrocytic anaemia

Causes of macrocytosis

Megaloblastic
- ○ B12 deficiency
- ○ Drugs, e.g. methotrexate
- ○ Folate deficiency

Non-megaloblastic (*mnemonic = MACRO*)
- ○ Myxoedema
- ○ Cirrhosis of the liver
- ○ Other: e.g. pregnancy, drugs
- ○ Alcohol excess
- ○ Reticulocytosis

Megaloblastic anaemias

Macrocytic anaemia with megaloblastic erythropoiesis in the bone marrow – increased size of all blood cell precursors particularly metamyelocytes (giant metamyelocytes). Blood film reveals macrocytic anaemia and hypersegmented neutrophils.

Causes of vitamin B12 deficiency

- ○ Inadequate dietary intake
- ○ Intrinsic factor deficiency: e.g. pernicious anaemia (autoimmune destruction of parietal cells or intrinsic factor), gastrectomy
- ○ Malabsorption: GI disease at terminal ileum, e.g. Crohn's disease, ileal resection

Complications of vitamin B12 deficiency include anaemia, peripheral neuropathy, subacute combined degeneration of the spinal cord, dementia. Diagnosis: based on low seum B12 levels; further tests include intrinsic factor and parietal cell antibodies and a Schilling test. Management: vitamin B12 deficiency can be treated with vitamin B12 injections or occasionally orally if cause is dietary deficiency.

Causes of folate deficiency

- ○ Inadequate dietary intake
- ○ Malabsorption
- ○ Increased requirement of folate: e.g. pregnancy, prematurity
- ○ Increased loss of folate: e.g. dialysis

DIAGNOSIS   Established by detecting reduced red cell folate levels. Treatment: replace folate orally.

10.11 Haemolytic anaemias

Causes of haemolytic anaemia

Inherited
○ Abnormality of red cell membrane: e.g. hereditary spherocytosis
○ Abnormality of the haemoglobin: e.g. sickle cell disease
○ Red cell enzyme defects: e.g. G6PD deficiency

Acquired
Immunologically mediated
○ Alloimmune: e.g. blood transfusion reaction, haemolytic disease of the newborn
○ Autoimmune: e.g. warm autoimmune haemolytic anaemia, paroxysmal cold haemoglobinuria, CHAD (cold haemagglutinin disease)

Non-immunological
○ Microangiopathic haemolytic anaemia (MAHA)
○ Infection: e.g. malaria
○ Prosthetic heart valves
○ Paroxysmal nocturnal haemoglobinaemia (PNH)

Increased red cell breakdown indicated by anaemia, reticulocytosis, raised unconjugated bilirubin, raised urinary urobilinogen, reduced haptoglobin, raised LDH. If intravascular haemolysis there may be haemoglobinuria, haemoglobinaemia; if extravascular there may be splenomegaly. Other tests to determine cause: blood film (e.g. sickle cells), direct anti-globulin test, Hb electrophoresis, enzyme assays.

Sickle cell disease
Autosomal recessive disorder, more common in black African population. Heterozygotes have sickle cell trait. Pathophysiology: abnormality of beta globin chains – when Hb deoxygenates, HbS molecules polymerise leading to sickle-shaped cells. Diagnosis: made on Hb electrophoresis.

COMPLICATIONS
● Vasoocclusive crises: infarction of bone due to blockage of small vessels causes pain. Precipitated by poor oxygenation, infection, dehydration. Treatment: rehydration, antibiotics if associated with infection, oxygen and analgesia.
● Aplastic crises: due to parvovirus, requires urgent transfusion.
● Sequestration crises: e.g. spleen, liver, may require urgent transfusion.
● Organ-threatening disease (e.g. chest) may require urgent exchange transfusion.

The thalassaemias
Reduced production of either alpha or beta globin chains leads to alpha and beta thalassaemia respectively. 'Major' if transfusion-dependent by one year of life, 'intermedia' and 'trait'. Diagnosis: severe microcytosis and hypochromia, Hb electrophoresis, raised HbA2 in beta thalassaemia. Treatment: blood transfusions which usually require associated iron chelation, e.g. with desferrioxamine.

10.12. Haematological emergencies
Neutropenic sepsis
MANAGEMENT
- Isolate the patient.
- Barrier nurse.
- Perform full septic screen (blood, urine, stool, sputum, chest x-ray).
- Treatment:
  - intravenous broad spectrum antibiotics without delay: usually local guidelines available and should be followed; close liason with microbiologist
  - consider fungal infection in patients with prolonged neutropenia
  - granulocyte colony stimulating factor (G-CSF) can be considered to increase the WCC.

See Endocrine section for treatment of hypercalcaemia.

10.13 Investigations
Blood film
An enormously useful and simple test. Gives information regarding morphology of red cells, white cells and platelets.

Bone marrow aspirate and trephine
Usually taken from the posterior superior iliac spine, occasionally from the sternum (or tibia in children only); provides important information regarding haematopoiesis and infiltration of bone marrow with abnormal cells. Aspirate fluid can also be sent as appropriate for cytogenetic testing, immunophenotyping and other relevant molecular markers, e.g. bcr-abl mutation in CML.

Oncology

11.1. Oncological treatments

Chemotherapy
Systemic treatment for cancer patients which may be administered IV, IM, intrathecally or orally.

Classes of chemotherapeutic agents.
- **Alkylating agents:** e.g. melphalan, chlorambucil, cyclophosphamide.
- **Platinum compounds:** e.g. cisplatin, carboplatin and oxaliplatin.
- **Antimetabolites:** e.g. methotrexate and 5-fluorouracil.
- **Anthracylines:** e.g. doxorubicin and bleomycin.
- **Topoisomerase inhibitors:** e.g. etoposide, topotecan.
- **Tubulin binding drugs:** e.g. vincristine, vinblastine, docetaxel.

Complications of chemotherapy

Acute: myelosuppression, nausea and vomiting, hair loss (alopecia), mouth ulceration

Delayed: cardiomyopathy (with doxorubicin), pulmonary fibrosis (with bleomycin), effects on spermatogenesis and oogenesis (patients should be offered the option to store semen and ovarian tissue), peripheral neuropathy

Hormone therapy
Growth of some tumours is 'hormone-dependent'; their cells express hormone receptors which can be targeted in treatment. Important examples include breast cancer – anti-oestrogens (e.g. tamoxifen) and aromatase inhibitors (e.g. exemestane); and prostate cancer – anti-androgens (e.g. zoladex).

Biological therapies
- **Active immunotherapy:** the aim is to elicit an immune reaction which can delay tumour growth, e.g. intravesical BCG in bladder cancer.
- **Monoclonal antibodies:** e.g. trastuzumab (Herceptin), a monoclonal antibody to HER-2 used in breast cancer.
- **Tyrosine kinase inhibitors:** e.g. Iressa, used in non-small cell lung cancer.

Radiotherapy
Radiosensitive tumours include oesophageal cancer, testicular seminoma, and lymphoma. Radiotherapy is also used for palliation in some tumours.

Brachytherapy is when a radioactive source in the form of beads or wires is implanted within or near tumour, e.g. Iridium192 used in prostate cancer.

Complications of radiotherapy

○ Skin erythema (common) +/– desquamation
○ Nausea and vomiting, diarrhoea
○ Oesophagitis: treat with soft diets and proton pump inhibitor
○ Mucositis
○ Radiation pneumonitis

11.2. Oncological emergencies

Spinal cord compression
See Neurology section

Hypercalcaemia
See Endocrinology section

Superior vena cava (SVC) obstruction
Occurs due to compression of the SVC by tumour/lymphadenopathy or more rarely by thrombus secondary to local involvement of the tumour.

CLINICAL FEATURES
● Breathlessness or stridor.
● Headache.
● Swelling of the face and arms, dysphagia.
● Dilated veins over the neck and chest.

MANAGEMENT
● Requires urgent imaging of the chest (CXR then CT).
● Treatment: dexamethasone acutely, radiotherapy (or chemotherapy if sensitive) +/– placement of a stent.

Neutropenic sepsis
Any patient who has had cytotoxic chemotherapy, which lowers the neutrophil count, is at risk of neutropenic sepsis.

MANAGEMENT   Full 'septic screen' (CXR, blood cultures, sputum/stool/urine cultures, lumbar puncture if indicated) to look for source. Treatment: broad spectrum antibiotics as per local protocol. If no response to antibiotics consider non-bacterial cause, e.g.fungal or viral. Isolate patient and barrier nurse.

11.3. Tumour markers
Substances produced by tumours, found in the blood. Concentrations found in peripheral blood decrease once the tumour is removed; thus concentration can be used as an indicator of tumour activity. Common tumour markers:
● CA125 – ovarian cancer (falsely elevated in liver disease and endometriosis).
● CA19-9 – upper gastrointestinal cancers, e.g. pancreatic cancer.
● CEA (carcinoembryonic antigen) – lower GI tract cancers.
● AFP – hepatocellular cancer.
● PSA – prostate cancer.
● Beta-HCG – choriocarcinoma.

12

Toxicology

12.1. Poisoning and overdose overview

When faced with any overdose (OD) or poisoning follow these general rules.

- Ask about timing of overdose, dose of drug taken, other drugs or alcohol use, suicidal intent, previous psychiatric history, HIV, hepatitis B or C status if relevant.
- Assess consciousness level (may need intubation), for cardiovascular stability and rhythm disturbance, respiratory depression, liver involvement.
- Investigations: paracetamol and salicylate levels, alcohol levels, U&Es, LFTs, FBC, clotting, ABGs, ECG, CXR, urine and blood toxicology screen.

Summary of management plan in poisoning/overdose

- Reduce absorption of drug: e.g. gastric lavage (rarely done now), activated charcoal (for certain drugs)
- Increase excretion: e.g. forced alkaline diuresis, haemodialysis (rarely required)
- Supportive measures: ABC, close observation, cardiac monitoring, fluids etc.
- Antidotes if available: e.g. naloxone for opiates
- Psychiatry review when medically fit (in intentional overdose setting)

Further information is available either from TOXBASE (computer database of poisoning management), or you can call the National Poisons Information Service.

12.2. Specific cases

Paracetamol

Follow the general rules as above.

- Timing of OD important: paracetamol levels should be performed at four hours post-OD as management is based on this result.
- Patients are classed as 'high risk' if alcoholic, on enzyme-inducing drugs, or have liver disease or HIV. The threshold for commencing specific treatment in these groups is lower as they have increased susceptibility.
- Treatment: N-acetylcysteine therapy is indicated if paracetamol levels are above the 'normal' or 'high risk' treatment lines on the normogram.
- Poor prognostic factors: raised INR, creatinine rise, and metabolic acidosis. May need to liaise with the regional liver unit.

Salicylates

Follow the general rules as above.

- Clinical features: tinnitus, nausea and vomiting; hyperventilation causing

respiratory alkalosis (stimulation of respiratory centre); metabolic acidosis; reduced GCS, hyperpyrexia and tachycardia. Watch for hypoglycaemia.
- Treatment: depends on salicylate levels at six hours; consider supportive care, alkaline diuresis, haemodialysis if large OD.

Opiates
Follow the general rules as above.
- Patients may be unconscious so no history available: look for pinpoint pupils and respiratory depression. Iatrogenic opiate overdose can occur following excess opiate administration post-surgery.
- Treatment: antidote is naloxone IV (improvement in conscious level is seen immediately +/− withdrawal symptoms but short-acting). Can also give IM as patients may abscond once they wake up, and the IM dose is longer-acting.

Benzodiazepines
Follow the general rules as above.
- Patients will be drowsy or unconscious, may have slurred speech, low blood pressure and slow heart rate. Respiratory depression occurs.
- Antidote is flumazenil, but only use if absolutely necessary. Patients often overdose on more than one drug and you may induce seizures if there are other drugs such as tricyclic antidepressants in the system.

Cocaine
Follow the general rules as above.
- Clinical features: tachycardia, chest pain, agitation, pyrexia, and convulsions.
- Management is supportive.

Amphetamines – Ecstasy
Follow the general rules as above.
- Clinical features: hyperpyrexia, confusion, convulsions, hallucinations, delirium, arrhythmias, rhabdomyolysis, renal failure, coagulopathy.
- Management is supportive.

Tricyclic antidepressants
Follow the general rules as above.
- Clinical features: neurological signs (dilated pupils, confusion, seizures) and cardiac signs (arrhythmias).
- Management is supportive; correct metabolic acidosis.

Carbon monoxide
Follow the general rules as above. Clue: flushed/red, headache, reduced GCS. Check carboxyhaemoglobin level (via ABG) and treat with high-flow oxygen.

Digoxin
Follow the general rules as above.
- Clinical features: nausea and vomiting, visual disturbances such as halos around objects and green/yellow vision, seizures, arrhythmias.
- Measure serum levels of digoxin.
- Management is supportive; prescribe digoxin-specific antibody (Fab) fragments if severe arrhythmia or haemodynamic instability, high serum digoxin levels, or significant overdose.

Surgery

13

General surgery

13.1. Obstructive jaundice

Also known as cholestatic jaundice; occurs as a result of obstruction within the extrahepatic or occasionally intrahepatic biliary trees. Observed clinically when serum bilirubin is >30 µmol/l.

Causes of obstructive jaundice

○ Extrahepatic: gallstones, malignancy (head of the pancreas, cholangiocarcinoma), primary sclerosing cholangitis, strictures, pancreatitis
○ Intrahepatic: cirrhosis, primary biliary cirrhosis, drugs (e.g. phenothiazines, oestrogens), malignancy (e.g. liver metastases)

CLINICAL FEATURES (DEPEND ON CAUSE)
- Jaundice, i.e. yellow pigmentation of skin, mucous membranes or cornea.
- May be painless, or present with colicky RUQ pain, depending on cause.
- Pruritis.
- Weight loss (cachexia) and anorexia.
- Ascites.
- Dark urine and steatorrhoea (due to fat malabsorption).
- Palpable gallbladder.

Courvoisier's Law: 'a palpable gallbladder (GB) and jaundice is unlikely to be due to gallstones (where the GB is shrunken and fibrotic)'; this usually indicates malignancy.

INVESTIGATIONS
- Blood tests: FBC (WCC increased in infection), U&Es, Clotting, Glucose.
- Liver function tests: increased ALP and GGT; raised (conjugated) bilirubin; normal/decreased albumin.
- Urinalysis (for conjugated bilirubin).
- Ultrasound: for calculi within gallbladder/duct, pancreatic mass, liver metastases, and common bile duct (CBD) diameter (if >8 mm suggests obstruction).
- AXR: unlikely to be helpful (shows <10% of gallstones).
- ERCP/MRCP +/– CT scan; liver biopsy may be necessary.

MANAGEMENT
- Fluid resuscitation.
- Analgesia: NSAIDs +/– pethidine (which relaxes the sphincter of Oddi); use opiates cautiously in liver failure.
- Antibiotics if infection: (Gram –ve cover; *Klebsiella, E. Coli, Enterococcus* sp. most commonly implicated pathogens).
- Correct coagulopathy (i.e. vitamin K or FFP).
- Antihistamines for pruritis.
- ERCP +/– stenting or sphincterotomy to relieve obstruction.
- Importantly, treat the underlying cause, e.g. laparoscopic or open cholecystectomy.

13.2. Gallbladder disease

PRESENTATION
- **Asymptomatic:** i.e. incidental finding ($\approx$ 85%).
- **Biliary colic:** (80% gallstones are mixed; 15% are pure cholesterol; 5% are pigmented stones).
  - Clinical features: recurrent, episodic colicky pain in RUQ, epigastrium or right shoulder tip (referred T5–7 pain) due to impaction of the stone at the GB neck; precipitated by eating fatty foods, and worse on inspiration; often associated with nausea, vomiting and anorexia.
- **Acute cholecystitis:** as above, with fever. Murphy's sign – pain on palpation of the RUQ, which is worse on inspiration, usually positive.
- **Obstructive jaundice**
  - Clinical features: jaundice, dark urine and steatorrhoea.
- **Ascending cholangitis:** *Charcot's triad* – fever/rigors, jaundice and RUQ pain.
- **GB perforation** (can be free or localised, usually occurs at the fundus due to gangrene of the GB) +/– **peritonitis** (seen with free perforation) +/– **gallstone ileus** (due to a localised perforation of the GB into the duodenum).
- **Pancreatitis.**
- **Empyema, mucocele:** due to gallstones impacting in Hartmann's pouch leading to obstruction to mucus flow and pain. Clinical features: palpable RUQ mass.

Predisposing factors to gallstones
- ○ Obesity
- ○ Terminal ileum disease: e.g. Crohn's due to malabsorption of bile salts
- ○ Cirrhosis
- ○ Haemolytic anaemia: e.g. sickle cell, hereditary spherocytosis (classically, pigmented stones)
- ○ Infections of the biliary tree: e.g. *E. Coli, Klebsiella* sp, *Streptococcus* sp.
- ○ Drugs: e.g. OCP, clofibrate, thiazide diuretics, long-term TPN

INVESTIGATIONS
- Blood tests: FBC (WCC increased in cholecystitis, cholangitis, pancreatitis), U&Es, clotting, LFTs, amylase (to exclude acute pancreatitis).
- Blood cultures.
- Urinalysis (for conjugated bilirubin).
- Erect CXR: to exclude perforated viscus.
- AXR: 10% gallstones radio-opaque; aerobilia (air within the biliary tree seen with gallstone ileus).
- Ultrasound.
  - Gallstones – sensitive for ≈ 95% GB stones and ≈ 80% CBD stones.
  - Thickened GB wall and pericholecystic fluid diagnostic of acute cholecystitis.
  - CBD dilation >8 mm suggests obstruction, i.e. stone/stricture.

MANAGEMENT
- Fluid resuscitation.
- Intravenous antibiotics (if evidence of infection).
- Analgesia.
- Correct coagulopathy.
- Dietary advice and weight loss.
- Interventional options.
  - ERCP/PTC (for CBD stones) +/– sphincterotomy +/– stenting (usually of a malignant stricture).
  - Open stone removal with T-tube insertion.
  - Delayed laparoscopic (or open) cholecystectomy – timing usually about six weeks post-acute episode, performed acutely in some centres.
- Other less common options.
  - Bile salts (however 50% recurrence of gallstones).
  - Extracorporeal shock wave lithotripsy (ESWL).

Complications of laparoscopic cholecystectomy

General
- ○ Associated with general anaesthesic (GA) or surgery in general, e.g. LRTI, PE, DVT

Specific
- ○ Damage to viscera (e.g. bowel or blood vessels – leading to bleeding) on port insertion
- ○ Complications of pneumoperitoneum: e.g. carbon dioxide embolus
- ○ Infection (e.g. wound)
- ○ Incisional or port-site hernia
- ○ CBD injury, bile leak
- ○ Conversion to an open procedure

Other diseases of the biliary system
Common bile duct/hepatic duct stricture
Clinical features: obstructive jaundice. Causes: iatrogenic; sclerosing cholangitis.

Gallbladder carcinoma
Clinical features: RUQ pain; jaundice; ascites; weight loss and anorexia. Poor prognosis (4% survival at five years).

Cholangiocarcinoma

Associated with CBD stones, UC and sclerosing cholangitis. Clinical features are similar to that of gallbladder carcinoma.

Choledochal cysts

Congenital; can lead to pancreatobiliary reflux. Clinical features: jaundice, RUQ pain and mass.

13.3. Splenic injury

Usually due to trauma – blunt or penetrating (Remember the spleen underlies the T9–11 ribs), or iatrogenic; spontaneous rupture can occur in splenomegaly.

CLINICAL FEATURES

- Left shoulder tip (referred) pain due to diaphragmatic irritation by blood/ haematoma.
- Shock (hypotension, tachycardia, cold, clammy peripheries).
- Tenderness or peritonism in the LUQ/flank.
- LUQ/flank bruising.
- Splenomegaly (NB: the spleen enlarges below the left costal margin towards the umbilicus; moves downwards with inspiration; has a palpable notch inferiorly and is dull to percussion unlike an enlarged left kidney).
- Regional lymph nodes and liver should be examined for enlargement.

INVESTIGATIONS

- Blood tests: urgent clotting, FBC, blood film, U&Es, LFTs, cross match six units of blood.
- CXR: for rib fractures.
- AXR: look for a displaced gastric bubble, soft tissue shadowing.
- CT scan with contrast (diagnostic).

MANAGEMENT

- Fluid resuscitation.
- Admit and observe in cases of trauma.
- Splenectomy is indicated in cases of:
  - rupture
  - malignancy
  - haematological disorders.
- Lifelong antibiotic cover post-splenectomy is controversial; vaccination against pnemococcus is however required.

COMPLICATIONS OF SPLENECTOMY

- Bleeding +/– shock.
- Thrombocytosis (risk DVT, PE; consider Aspirin).
- Sepsis, LRTI (atelectasis) + subphrenic abscess.

13.4. Pancreatic disease

Acute pancreatitis

Acute inflammation of the pancreas. Peak incidence: 40–50 years. Men and women equally affected.

Causes of acute pancreatitis

The classic mnemonic is 'GET SMASHED' but note that 15% are idiopathic
- Gallstones (45%)
- Ethanol (25%)

Other causes are rare:
- Trauma, post renal or cardiac transplant; Steroids; Mumps; Autoimmune; Scorpion venom (rare!); Hyperlipidaemia, hypercalcaemia; ERCP (4%); Drugs, e.g. thiazide diuretics, fibrates

CLINICAL FEATURES
- Epigastric pain radiating to the back with associated nausea, vomiting, anorexia +/– obstructive jaundice.
- Dehydration.
- Tenderness +/– guarding in the epigastrium + decreased/absent bowel sounds.
- Grey-Turner's sign: blood tracking into the left paracolic gutter (flank).
- Cullen's sign: periumbilical echymoses.

INVESTIGATIONS
- Blood tests: FBC (WCC increased in inflammation), CRP (prognostic indicator in first 48 hours and useful for monitoring disease), U&Es, LFTs, serum glucose (hyperglycaemia due to destruction of β-islet cells), clotting, serum calcium, arterial blood gas.
- Amylase >1000 U/l or 4× normal is diagnostic; falls after 24 hours; serum lipase.
- Blood cultures.
- Erect CXR: to exclude perforation, ARDS, effusion.
- AXR: for loss of psoas shadow, ileus, calcified head of pancreas (suggests chronic pathology).
- Ultrasound gallbladder: for gallstones (cause).
- CT abdomen: for necrosis and haemorrhage.
- Disease is scored as mild, moderate or severe using predictive criteria, e.g. Ranson's or the modified Glasgow criteria.

Glasgow scoring system *(mnemonic = 'PANCREAS')*

P – PaO$_2$ <8 kPa
A – Age >55 years
N – Neutrophilia, i.e. WCC >15×10^9/l
C – Calcium <2 mmol/l
R – Renal function: Urea >16 mmol/l
E – Enzymes: LDH>600 U/l
A – AST/ALT >200 U/l
S – Sugar, i.e. Glucose >10 mmol/ml

The presence of three or more factors within the first 48 hours suggests severe pancreatitis.

MANAGEMENT
- Transfer to ITU/HDU as appropriate.
- Oxygen therapy and respiratory support as necessary.
- Keep NBM, i.e. rest pancreas, NG tube for drainage of stomach contents.
- Insert urinary catheter and fluid resuscitate; consider CVP line insertion to guide fluid regimen.

- Analgesia.
- Medical treatment includes:
  - antibiotics – if infection (Gram and anaerobic cover); prophylactic use is controversial
  - correct electrolytes: e.g. hypocalcaemia, hypomagnesaemia
  - sliding scale insulin
  - consider TPN/NJ feeding after five days of NBM.
- Treat underlying cause, e.g. gallstones with cholecystectomy, alcoholism with rehabilitation.
- Surgery: indicated for complications, e.g. pancreatic necrosis or abscess, pseudocyst.

Complications of acute pancreatitis

- Sepsis, SIRS (Systemic Inflammatory Response Syndrome), ARDS (Adult Respiratory Distress Syndrome), MODS (Multi-Organ Dysfunction Syndrome)
- Hypocalcaemia, Hypomagnesaemia
- Hyperglycaemia (diabetes)
- Pancreatic necrosis
- Pancreatic pseudocysts or abscess or haemorrhage
- Chronic pancreatitis
- Splenic vein thrombosis
- Death (5–10%)

Chronic pancreatitis
Irreversible pancreatic inflammation characterised by chronic pain requiring opiate analgesia, and pancreatic atrophy with loss of exocrine and endocrine function. Associated with an increased risk of pancreatic carcinoma. Peak incidence 35–45 years.

Causes of chronic pancreatitis

- Alcohol (70%)
- Obstruction, i.e. ductal strictures, gallstones, tumours, pancreatic divisum
- Metabolic: hypercalcaemia, hyperlipidaemia
- Cystic Fibrosis
- Radiation
- Idiopathic (30%)

Clinical features: classically, chronic epigastric pain radiating into the back with acute severe episodes; associated nausea, weight loss, polydipsia and polyuria (diabetes) and steatorrhoea (due to fat malabsorption); cachexia, epigastric tenderness +/– abdominal mass +/– jaundice (if pseudocysts develop).

INVESTIGATIONS
- Serum amylase, lipase and CRP usually normal.
- Blood glucose (for diabetes); GGT (for alcohol excess).
- Abdominal x-ray (may show a calcified pancreas).
- Ultrasound (for dilated CBD or gallstones).
- Abdominal CT scan (for complications, i.e. cysts, abscess, necrosis) +/– ERCP.
- Pancreatic function tests, i.e. Lundh, pancreolauryl test, rarely used.

MANAGEMENT
- Keep NBM – rest pancreas, IV fluids, NG tube, analgesia +/– TPN or NJ feeding in the acute phase.
- Treat underlying cause: e.g. help with stopping alcohol.
- Chronic pain management – refer to pain team.
- Treat metabolic complications: diabetes control; pancreatic enzyme and vitamin supplements; proton pump inhibitor.
- Surgery: to relieve obstruction, for intractable pain or failed conservative treatment.

Cancer of the pancreas
- More common in men.
- Risk factors: smoking; chronic pancreatitis, carcinogens.
- Pathology: ≈ 90% ductal adenocarcinoma.
- Spread: direct extension to CBD, duodenum, blood vessels, stomach and spleen; lymphatic and haematogenous to liver and lungs.
- Prognosis is poor: five year survival <2%.

CLINICAL FEATURES
- Weight loss, anorexia.
- Epigastric pain – radiating to the back.
- Painless obstructive jaundice.
- Diabetes.
- On examination: cachexia, jaundice, epigastric tenderness +/– epigastric mass, ascites.

INVESTIGATIONS
- Blood tests: FBC (for anaemia), U&Es, LFTs (for obstructive jaundice), clotting, glucose, CA19-9 (90% sensitive).
- Staging: CXR, CT scan +/– laparoscopy +/– endoluminal ultrasound.

MANAGEMENT
- Treat jaundice: prurutis with anti-histamines; ERCP +/– stenting to relieve obstruction.
- Surgery: e.g. Whipples's procedure, distal pancreatectomy.
- Palliation: control pain (opiate analgesia, coeliac plexus block, radiotherapy); involve palliative care team.

13.5. The acute abdomen
Pain in the abdomen of acute (<1 week) duration, with associated symptoms, e.g. anorexia, nausea, vomiting, change in bowel habits, jaundice, fever and urinary or gynaecological symptoms.

Diagnosis relies on a comprehensive history, examination and focussed investigations. On examination, there is tenderness of the abdomen (+/– rebound or percussion tenderness) with or without abdominal distension, guarding and decreased or absent bowel sounds. In addition, there may be signs of dehydration and sepsis.

Differential diagnosis depends on the site of pain
The abdomen can be divided into nine regions (see diagram) or four quadrants:

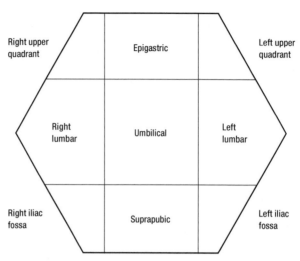

FIGURE 13.1 Differential diagnosis depends on site of pain.

Differential diagnosis of pain dependent on site

Epigastric
- GI: acute +/− chronic pancreatitis, biliary colic; acute cholecystitis, peptic ulcer disease, perforation
- Vascular: ruptured AAA
- Cardiac: myocardial infarction

Right Upper Quadrant (RUQ)
- GI: biliary colic, acute cholecystitis, cholangitis, hepatitis
- Respiratory: lower lobe pneumonia, subphrenic abscess
- Urological: renal colic, pyelonephritis

Left Upper Quadrant (LUQ)
- GI: splenic pathology, acute +/− chronic pancreatitis
- Respiratory: lower lobe pneumonia

Right Iliac Fossa (RIF)
- GI: acute appendicitis, Meckel's diverticulitis, mesenteric adenitis, caecal carcinoma (consider in older patients), perforation, carcinoid tumour, IBD
- Gynaecological causes: Pelvic Inflammatory Disease (PID); ruptured ovarian cyst; torsion fallopian tubes; ectopic pregnancy
- Urological causes: ureteric colic, pyelonephritis

Left Iliac Fossa (LIF)
- GI causes: diverticulitis
- Gynaecological causes: ectopic pregnancy; torsion fallopian tubes; PID; ruptured ovarian cyst
- Urological causes: ureteric colic, pyelonephritis

Suprapubic
- Urological causes: cystitis; UTI; acute urinary retention
- Gynaecological causes

INVESTIGATIONS
- Blood tests: FBC, clotting, group and save, U&Es, LFTs, amylase, CRP, blood cultures.
- Urinalysis (includes β-HCG to exclude pregnancy).
- ABG.
- Erect CXR (to exclude pneumonia, free air under diaphragm with perforation).
- AXR (for intestinal obstruction or renal calculi).
- Further imaging: ultrasound, CT scanning (+/– contrast).

MANAGEMENT   Tailored to the cause but may include: NBM, IV fluid resuscitation, NG tube insertion, analgesia, antibiotics (once diagnosis established); watchful waiting or surgery (open or laparoscopic).

Peritonitis – *inflammation of the peritoneum*
This can be classified as *generalised* or *localised*; and *primary* (i.e. spontaneous or due to peritoneal dialysis) or *secondary* to pathology elsewhere, e.g. acute appendicitis. Pain in peritonitis is typically localised, due to the somatic innervation of the parietal peritoneum. In contrast, visceral pain (ANS innervation) is poorly localised and often referred to specific dermatomes, i.e. referred pain.

13.6. Acute appendicitis
Inflammation of the appendix. Pathologically: luminal obstruction due to lymphoid hyperplasia following a viral infection or obstruction due to a faecolith.

FEATURES IN THE HISTORY
- Peak incidence in childhood (rare prior to two years).
- Pain: initially colicky and periumbilical (T10), becoming constant and localising to the RIF; worse with movement.
- Nausea and occasionally vomiting, anorexia.

FEATURES ON EXAMINATION
- Low grade fever, fetor oris, tachycardia.
- Tenderness RIF (maximal at McBurney's point – located one third of the distance from the anterior superior iliac spine (ASIS) to the umbilicus); guarding +/– rebound and/or percussion tenderness.
- Rovsing's sign: pain in RIF on palpation of the LIF.
- Psoas sign: pain on thigh extension (due to inflammation adjacent to the psoas muscle).
- Rarely, tender mass in RIF (in elderly, be cautious as likely caecal tumour).
- Tender PR examination (suggests a pelvic appendix).

INVESTIGATIONS
- Blood tests: FBC (increased WCC in inflammation and infection); U&Es, CRP, clotting, group and save.
- Urinalysis to exclude UTI (nitrites) or renal stones (haematuria).
- β-HCG to exclude pregnancy/ectopic pregnancy.
- Ultrasound (useful for excluding pelvic pathology; less sensitive for appendicitis).

MANAGEMENT
- Fluid resuscitation and keep NBM.
- Analgesia.
- Give antibiotics only once diagnosis is established.
- Laparoscopic or open appendicectomy (via modified Lanz/grid-iron incision).
- If appendiceal mass – interval appendicectomy; treat with antibiotics.

Complications of appendicitis
- Mural necrosis/gangrene and perforation
- Peritonitis
- Paralytic ileus
- Abscess
- Post-operatively: wound infection; intra-abdominal/pelvic abscess

13.7. Disorders of the small bowel

Tumours
Account for 3–6% of all GI tumours. Can be *primary* or *secondary*, e.g. due to peritoneal seeding or malignant melanoma. Clinical features: can present with haemorrhage, intussusception or obstruction. Investigations: AXR, barium follow-through (for strictures, tumours, mucosal defects); upper and lower GI endoscopy +/–biopsy; red cell scanning (for a source of bleeding); staging CT scan.

Primary small bowel tumours

Benign: lipoma, fibroma, leiomyoma, neurofibroma, adenoma, carcinoid <2 cm

Malignant: adenocarcinoma, carcinoid >2 cm + liver spread, lymphoma (B or T-cell)

Carcinoid tumours and syndrome
Tumour of APUD (amine precursor uptake) system. Majority occur in GI tract (appendix and ileum most common sites). If >2 cm increased risk of malignancy. Clinical features: 1% develop carcinoid syndrome: flushing, diarrhoea and bronchospasm due to serotonin release from metastatic disease. Investigations: as above, in addition, perform urinalysis for 5-hydroxyindoleacetate (5-HIAA). Treatment: octreotide (somatostatin analogue) or surgical resection/embolisation of liver metastases and the primary lesion.

Meckel's diverticulum
Congenital diverticulum lined with intestinal or ectopic gastric or pancreatic mucosa. Embryological remnant of vitello-intestinal duct. Rule of 2s: persists in 2% of the population; is two inches long and is found two feet from the ileocaecal valve. Clinical features: majority asymptomatic; often an incidental finding at surgery. Complications include inflammation (pain mimics appendicitis), peptic ulceration and bleeding +/– perforation, intussusception, volvulus or obstruction. Investigations: Meckel's technetium scan or barium follow-through. Treatment: surgical resection if symptomatic.

Intussusception
Invagination/prolapse of a segment of bowel through its own lumen. The invaginated bowel is termed the *intussusceptum*. Aetiology: 95% of cases occur in children/ infants. In adults, a tumour more commonly forms the apex of the intussusceptum. More common in males. Clinical features: colicky abdominal pain; vomiting which may be faeculent; 'redcurrant jelly' stools. Occasionally the intussusceptum

is palpable – so-called epigastric 'tumour' (mass). DRE reveals 'redcurrant jelly'. Complications include strangulation, gangrene and peritonitis. Management: hydrostatic reduction with barium enema (also diagnostic); surgical reduction or bowel resection if gangrene. Note that there is a high incidence of recurrence.

13.8. Intestinal obstruction

Obstruction can be *mechanical* or *non-mechanical* (ileus or pseudo-obstruction). Complications include strangulation; gangrene; perforation and peritonitis.

Causes of small bowel obstruction (SBO) – *most common causes numbered 1–4*

- ○ **Extrinsic:** hernias (1), adhesions (2), volvulus, compression by mass/abscess
- ○ **Intramural:** Crohn's disease (3), tumour (4), intussusception, stricture, atresia
- ○ **Intraluminal:** foreign body, gallstones, faecolith, phyto- or trichobezoar, meconium
- ○ **Causes of large bowel obstruction (LBO):** colon carcinoma (70%), hernias, volvulus (sigmoid or caecal), Crohn's disease, stricture

CLINICAL FEATURES
- Colicky abdominal pain (central in SBO; RIF if ileocaecal valve is competent).
- Vomiting (faeculent, occurring early in high obstructions).
- Absolute constipation (no flatus/faeces); associated abdominal distension.
- Other: sepsis (suggests strangulation); scars (points to adhesions as the cause) or hernias; hyperactive bowel sounds (decreased/absent in pseudo-obstruction); empty rectum on DRE.

INVESTIGATIONS
- Blood tests: FBC (increased WCC in inflammation and infection), U&Es (assess hydration), Mg^{2+}, LFTs, clotting, Group and Save and arterial blood gas.
- AXR: In SBO small bowel is dilated >3 cm (*small bowel can be identified by valvulae conniventes and central position*); in LBO large bowel may be dilated to >6 cm and the caecum to >9 cm (*large bowel can be identified by the presence of haustra and peripheral position*).
- Gastrograffin follow-through, enema (for pseudo-obstruction).

MANAGEMENT
- 'Drip and suck': fluid resuscitation, keep NBM, insert NG tube and give analgesia.
- In SBO, if no evidence of strangulation, observe for resolution. Surgery indicated if SBO fails to resolve within 24 hours or strangulation.
- In LBO, obstruction may be relieved with a deflatus tube. Surgery is indicated if the caecum is >10 cm (suggesting imminent risk of perforation).
- Investigate cause, e.g. CT if malignancy suspected.

Pseudo-obstruction

Non-mechanical bowel obstruction. Causes: metabolic (e.g. high K^+, low Na^+, low Ca^{2+}), drugs (e.g. opiates), neurological and idiopathic.

Clinical features: gradual painless abdominal distension and constipation. Tympanic, non-tender abdomen with decreased/absent bowel sounds.

Management: 'Drip and suck,' rehydrate and correct electrolyte imbalance. Decompress by colonoscopy if the diameter of the large bowel is >9 cm due to increased risk of perforation. Prokinetic agents may be helpful, e.g. neostigmine, erythromycin. Usually self-limiting. Surgery is indicated if conservative treatment fails.

13.9. Ischaemic bowel

A reduction in the blood supply to the small bowel (mesenteric ischaemia), large bowel (ischaemic colitis), or less commonly both, resulting in ischaemia, infarction (+/– perforation), sepsis, and eventually death. Onset can be *acute* or *chronic*.

Causes of ischaemic bowel

Hypoperfusion due to decreased cardiac output:
- Shock (e.g. septic, hypovolaemic)
- Cardiac disease, i.e. CCF, MI

Occlusion of the blood supply, in the absence of a sufficient collateral blood supply to maintain bowel wall integrity:
- Arterial thrombosis
- Venous thrombosis: risk factors include polycythaemia, thrombophilia, malignancy
- Embolus: e.g. cardiac following MI or with AF
- Vasculitis
- Fibromuscular dysplasia
- Aortic dissection
- Adhesions, hernia and volvulus

CLINICAL FEATURES *Mesenteric ischaemia:* diffuse colicky pain, onset is gradual in thrombosis, sudden if embolus; associated with nausea, vomiting, fever +/– diarrhoea. *Ischaemic colitis:* typically left-sided abdominal pain; associated with fever and bloody diarrhoea. Often a history of previous similar episodes and risk factors for vascular disease. In chronic disease, pain is typically worse with eating and relieved with opening bowels. Atherosclerosis is commonly implicated.

FEATURES ON EXAMINATION Abdominal distension and tenderness progressing to peritonitis, i.e. guarding, rebound/percussion tenderness, absent bowel sounds. Often patient is dehydrated.

INVESTIGATIONS
- Blood tests: FBC (raised WCC), ABG (severe lactic/metabolic acidosis – often occurs late).
- AXR may show obstruction; erect CXR to exclude perforation.
- Further imaging to aid diagnosis of cause: Doppler US, CT, MRA and mesenteric angiography; colonoscopy (for strictures/ulceration), and barium enema (for pathopneumonic 'thumb-printing') for ischaemic colitis.

MANAGEMENT ABC, fluid resuscitation, NBM, NG tube, IV antibiotics. Treat precipitating cause. Surgery: resection if infarction +/– stoma; embolectomy; revascularisation +/– thrombolysis. Palliation in select cases.

13.10. Diverticular disease

Outpouchings from the colonic lumen due to herniation of mucosa and submucosa through '*points of weakness*' in the bowel wall, i.e. at sites of entry of nutrient blood vessels. Commonly affects the distal colon with sigmoid involved in 90% of cases. More common with increasing age affects: 5–10% under 40 years; 30% >60 years; 50% >70 years. More common in males and in developed countries. Associated with a low fibre diet and increasing age. Predisposing factors are obesity, immobility, caffeine and alcohol intake, cigarette smoking, polycystic kidney disease, and mixed connective tissue disorders.

CLINICAL FEATURES
- Usually asymptomatic but occasionally, colicky abdominal pain, bloating flatulence, constipation/diarrhoea and LIF tenderness; symptoms typically improve with opening bowels or passage of flatus.
- ≈ 20% develop complications.

Complications of diverticular disease

○ **Acute diverticulitis:** inflammation in one or more diverticula. Clinical features: LIF (or less commonly RIF) pain, anorexia, nausea and vomiting +/– change in bowel habit +/– urinary symptoms (due to proximity of the sigmoid colon to the bladder); may have palpable mass on abdominal exam; DRE – mass/tenderness
○ **Peritonitis secondary to perforation**
○ **Obstruction**
○ **Strictures**
○ **Diverticular fistula:** pneumaturia/faecouria indicates a colovesical fistula; colovaginal fistula are more common post-hysterectomy
○ **PR Bleeding**

INVESTIGATIONS
- Blood tests: FBC (raised WCC but may be absent in immunosuppressed, elderly).
- Erect CXR (free gas under the diaphragm in perforation).
- AXR +/– gastrograffin (for dilated bowel in obstruction/ileus). *Avoid barium due to the risk of chemical peritonitis with extravasation of barium into the peritoneal cavity.*
- Ultrasound (for abscess).
- CT scanning with contrast (useful first line diagnostic test).

MANAGEMENT
- Conservative: fluid resuscitation, rest bowel (NBM or clear fluids orally), analgesia, IV antibiotics (e.g. cefuroxime + metronidazole), gradual introduction of oral intake with evidence of recovery. Long term: high fibre diet.
- Surgical: manage complications, e.g. CT/ultrasound-guided or open drainage of abscess; resection of diseased segment, e.g. Hartmann's procedure.

Hirschsprung's disease

Aganglionosis of the myenteric (Auerbach's) and Meissner's submucosal plexi. Recto-sigmoid junction involved in 80% of cases; small bowel can also be affected. Clinical features: classically presents with the delayed passage of meconium in first 24 hours after birth +/– abdominal distension and bilious vomiting.

13.11. Tumours of the large bowel

Polyps

Can be *neoplastic* or *non-neoplastic,* i.e. hyperplastic, harmartomatous polyps. Neoplastic polyps can be morphologically classified as either sessile or pedunculated; three histological types:
○ **Tubular adenoma:** most common benign polyp; <5% malignant; often pedunculated; diameter usually <2.5 cm. Risk of malignant change increases with increasing size

○ **Villous adenoma:** higher likelihood of malignant change (≈ 40%); usually sessile and large
○ **Tubulovillous adenoma:** features of both; intermediate risk of malignant change

Colorectal cancer

Second most common cause of cancer-related death in men (after lung cancer) in developed world. Third most common cause in women, after breast and lung cancer. Male to Female ratio 2:1. Peak incidence 60–70 years

Risk factors

- Increasing age: >50 years.
- Low fibre diet (increased transit time).
- High intake saturated fats + red meat.
- Increased faecal bile salts.
- Smoking.
- IBD (particularly UC).
- Previous colorectal cancer.
- Genetic predisposition.
- Familial adenomatous polyposis (FAP): mutation in APC gene.
- Gardener's syndrome: variant of FAP with osteomas, epidermal cysts, fibromatosis.
- Hereditary non-polyposis colon cancer (HNPCC).

≈ 98% are adenocarcinomas arising from pre-existing adenomatous polyps, i.e. adenoma-carcinoma sequence. Spread can be local, lymphatic and haematogenous to regional lymph nodes, liver, lungs and bone. Distribution: 50% occur in the rectum; 25% in the sigmoid colon; 12.5% in the caecum and descending colon; 12.5% at other sites. Synchronous lesions are present in 2–5% of cases.

CLINICAL FEATURES

- Occult blood loss with weight loss, fatigue, and anaemia – typically occur with right-sided tumours.
- Obstruction, colicky abdominal pain, distension, altered bowel habit +/– anorexia and nausea (vomiting occurs late) – more common with left-sided lesions.
- In rectal cancers: fresh PR bleeding, tenesmus and anal pain.
- Family history of FAP, colon cancer and UC should also be elicited.
- Examination is usually unremarkable in early disease. Cachexia, abdominal pain and distension, hepatomegaly, ascites and the presence of an abdominal mass are late signs. DRE may reveal a rectal mass, bleeding or occult blood.

INVESTIGATIONS

- Blood tests: FBC (microcytic anaemia); liver function tests (for liver metastases); alkaline phosphatase and serum calcium (increased if bony metastases).
- Faecal occult blood (FOB).
- Carcinoembryonic antigen (CEA): sensitive but not specific – elevated in colon cancer, pancreatic and hepatobiliary disease; useful for assessing response to treatment and recurrence.
- Colonoscopy/barium enema (*may see 'apple core lesion'*).
- CXR (for lung metastases + assess fitness for surgery).
- Endo-/transrectal ultrasound (first line for local staging of rectal carcinoma).
- CT scanning (useful for assessing spread to liver and LN and complications).

- MRI (useful in rectal carcinoma to determine local spread).
- PET (used to assess recurrence).

Prognosis

Depends on the pathological stage: modified Dukes-Bussey (D-B) staging system and TMN classification are the most widely used.

D-B staging system five-year survival:

Stage A	Tumour within wall; not penetrating muscularis propria; LN not involved	95%
Stage B	Tumour penetrating muscularis propria into extramural tissue; LN not involved	75%
Stage C1	Spread to regional LN	40%
Stage C2	Spread to regional LN with highest/apical node involvement	10%

TREATMENT   Depends on stage.
- Curative surgical resection for early disease + adjuvant chemotherapy (if LN involvement).
- Palliative surgery or chemotherapy in metastatic disease.
- Radiotherapy to reduce recurrence in rectal cancer and for palliation of bony pain.

Note: In individuals with FAP the risk of developing colorectal cancer is 100% (mean age 39 years) and a prophylactic total colectomy at age 20–30 years is recommended.

Screening for colorectal cancer

Screening can reduce the risk of death from bowel cancer by ≈ 16%. By 2009, the NHS Bowel Cancer Screening Programme will be fully operational. Men and women aged 60–69 years old will be routinely screened every two years using FOB testing kits. Those >70 years can request to be screened. Abnormal results will be investigated with colonoscopy.

13.12. Abdominal wall hernia

A hernia is an abnormal protrusion of all or part of a viscus through a defect in the wall of the cavity that normally contains it. Complications: incarceration, obstruction or strangulation (a Richter's hernia is a strangulated but not obstructed hernia).

Inguinal: the most common type (*see* below).

Femoral: protrusion of a viscus through the femoral canal. More common in women. On examination, hernia originates below the inguinal ligament and lateral to the pubic tubercle. High risk of obstruction/strangulation and therefore management is surgical.

Incisional: due to an acquired weakness, usually iatrogenic (affects 6% of abdominal wounds at five years) or traumatic. Hernia may become irreducible and can cause intestinal obstruction/strangulation of the contents of the hernia sac. Management: conservative or surgical (via a mesh repair, Keel (Maingot) repair, or layer-to-layer repair); can be repaired laparoscopically.

Para-umbilical: an acquired hernia due to a defect in the linea alba. Associated with obesity, ascites, pregnancy and increasing age. Equal incidence in men and women. Complications: intestinal obstruction/strangulation.

Umbilical: true umbilical herniae are congenital (as a consequence of abnormalities in development of the abdominal wall, e.g. exomphalos or gastroschisis).

Epigastric: defect in the linea alba resulting in usually a pea-sized lump.

Spigellian: herniation which occurs between the semilunar line and lateral border of the rectus sheath. Accounts for <1% of all hernias. Presence usually confirmed with ultrasound.

Obturator: protrusion of peritoneum through the obturator canal. Rare.

Lumbar: may be primary, resulting in a hernia through the superior or the inferior lumbar triangle of Petit, or acquired, i.e. post renal surgery.

Inguinal hernia
Incidence: higher in men than women (ratio 9:1) and increases with age. Possibly congenital due to a patent processus vaginalis or acquired. More common on the right than the left, thought to be due to the later descent of the testes on this side and to structural weakening post-appendicectomy.

Risk factors for acquired herniae
- Causes of increased intra-abdominal pressure: smoking (due to chronic cough), COPD, occupation (i.e. lifting), chronic constipation, benign prostate hyperplasia (BPH).
- Causes of a weakened abdominal wall: obesity, ilio-inguinal nerve damage, ascites and collagen disorders.

Anatomy of the inguinal canal
The inguinal canal extends from the deep inguinal ring (midpoint of the inguinal ligament) to the superficial ring (at the pubic tubercle). The boundaries include:
- ○ **Anterior wall:** external oblique aponeurosis + fibres of internal oblique laterally
- ○ **Roof:** fibres of internal oblique
- ○ **Floor:** inguinal ligament
- ○ **Posterior wall:** fascia transversalis + conjoint tendon medially

The contents of the inguinal canal include the spermatic cord + ilio-inguinal nerve.

CLINICAL FEATURES
- Lump in the groin, originating above the inguinal ligament and medial to the pubic tubercle, which transmits a cough impulse; may be reducible (i.e. the hernia sac can be returned to its containing cavity) or irreducible (incarcerated).
- Classified as direct or indirect: direct hernia lie medial to (i.e. passes through Hasselbach's triangle) and indirect hernia lie lateral to the inferior epigastric artery.
- Indirect hernia may be controlled with pressure over the deep inguinal ring.
- Lump typically enlarges with coughing, straining or crying (in children).
- Strangulation/obstruction suggested by presence of an irreducible, tense and tender lump, pain, vomiting, absolute constipation +/– decreased bowel sounds +/– associated skin changes.
- Diagnosis is clinical. Rarely ultrasound, herniography or CT is indicated.

Differential diagnosis of a groin lump

- ○ Inguinal/femoral hernia
- ○ Hydrocele of the spermatic cord
- ○ Inguinal lymphadenopathy
- ○ Lipoma of the cord or femoral canal
- ○ Iliofemoral aneurysm
- ○ Sapheno-varix
- ○ Psoas abscess
- ○ Undescended/ectopic testes

MANAGEMENT

- **Conservative:** Risk factor modification, i.e. weight loss, smoking cessation, treatment of constipation. If unfit/refuses surgery a well-fitting truss may be beneficial.
- **Surgical:** Repair can be performed in a daycase setting either laparoscopically (using mesh), or via an open approach (Lichtenstein (tension-free mesh), Shouldice, McVay and Bassini repairs). Open repair can be performed under a local or general anaesthetic. Complications of open hernia repair may be *immediate* (haematoma), *early* (infection, ischaemic orchitis), or *late* (recurrence – 2%, ilio-inguinal nerve damage).

13.13. Lower gastrointestinal bleeding

Defined as blood loss from a site distal to the ligament of Treitz. The majority of cases originate from the large bowel. Approximately 90% will cease spontaneously.

Causes of lower GI bleeding

- ○ **Diverticular disease:** risk of bleeding ≈ 15%; accounts for 40% of all lower GI bleeds; usually brisk and bright red
- ○ **Angiodysplasia:** bleeding classically intermittent; lesions are usually right-sided and multiple. Diagnosis and treatment is with angiography and embolisation acutely; colonoscopy may reveal 'cherry-red' areas and dilated tortuous vessels
- ○ **Ischaemic colitis:** usually affects the splenic flexure; commonly dark red bleeding associated with abdominal pain, distension and diarrhoea
- ○ **Inflammatory bowel disease:** proctitis or colitis; typically bloody diarrhoea
- ○ **Colorectal neoplasia:** right-sided lesions – typically chronic occult blood loss resulting in anaemia. Left-sided lesions – typically bright red PR blood, mixed with the stool
- ○ **Haemorrhoids** (*see* perianal disease)
- ○ **Meckel's diverticulum:** ectopic gastric mucosa within a Meckel's can ulcerate and bleed (commonly dark red blood)
- ○ **Other:** radiation proctocolitis, haemangiomas, iatrogenic, i.e. post-polypectomy, clotting abnormalities

CLINICAL FEATURES

- Colour of blood: bright red implies source is from rectum/anus; mixed/dark red suggests bleed is from the lower one-third of the bowel; melaena (black tarry stool) suggests an upper GI bleed.
- Duration and volume of blood loss gives an indication of the severity of the bleed. In addition, associated symptoms of weight loss, change in bowel habit, abdominal pain, tenesmus and diarrhoea will aid diagnosis.

MANAGEMENT
- ABC, IV access + fluid resuscitation, catheterise and monitor fluid balance closely.
- Urgent blood tests for FBC, U&Es, clotting. Cross-match four units of blood.
- DRE and proctosigmoidoscopy to exclude a distal source.
- OGD if blood loss is massive to exclude an upper GI bleed.
- Splanchnic angiography +/– adrenaline or embolisation of the bleeding vessel.
- 99m technetium red cell scanning (useful if blood loss is intermittent).
- Colonoscopy: technically difficult in the acute setting in an unprepared bowel.
- Surgery +/– on-table enteroscopy is indicated if blood loss is profuse and life-threatening, and an upper GI cause has been excluded.

13.14. Disorders of the rectum and anus
Fistula-in-ano
An abnormal communication between skin of the perineum and the anorectal canal. Classified according to its site, as: inter-, trans-, supra- or extrasphincteric. Incidence is 2–4 times higher in men; mean age of onset 40 years. Causes: infection of anal glands/crypts, IBD, hidradenitis suppurativa, malignancy (rectal/anal).

CLINICAL FEATURES
- Perianal or ischiorectal pain +/– perianal discharge.
- History of previous perianal abscess drainage or IBD.
- Examine for induration of the perianal skin to locate the primary tract; the internal opening may be palpated on DRE.

INVESTIGATIONS MRI (useful for complex fistulae); ultrasound/fistulography (superseded by MRI).

TREATMENT
- Emergency abscess drainage under GA + rigid sigmoidoscopy (to exclude IBD).
- Elective examination under anaesthetic (EUA) to define fistula anatomy with laying open of fistula tract (+ sphincter repair), seton or fibrin glue.

Goodsall's rule
If the external opening lies anterior to an imaginary line between 3.00 and 9.00 o'clock, the internal opening will lie anteriorly in the anal canal. If the external opening lies posterior, the internal opening will lie in the midline posteriorly.

Pilonidal sinus
A subcutaneous, hair-containing sinus tract. Typically occurs in young, hairy males (male to female ratio 4:1) at the natal cleft; can occur in the interdigital folds (in barbers/animal groomers), axilla or umbilicus.

CLINICAL FEATURES Usually presents with localised pain, mass, tenderness and discharge due to pilonidal abscess. Management: analgesia, incision and drainage of the abscess acutely; followed by elective excision of the sinus.

Perianal abscess
Infection of the soft tissue surrounding the anal canal, often associated with a fistulous tract. Thought to arise from infection of the anal glands/crypts lining the anal canal; E.coli, *Enterococcus* sp. and *Bacteroides* sp. commonly implicated.

More common in men (2–3 ×). Classified according to location as *perianal* (60%), *ischiorectal* (20%), *intersphincteric* (5%), *supralevator* and *submucosal*.

CLINICAL FEATURES   Presents as a fluctuant perianal mass, perianal discomfort, erythema, purulent discharge, pruritus +/– fever; 30% describe previous episodes.

MANAGEMENT   Bacterial wound swab + incision and drainage of abscess under GA. Exclude diabetes mellitus.

Anal fissure
A tear in the squamous epithelium of the distal anal canal. Usually occurs posteriorly; can be acute or chronic (>6 weeks duration). Common in young adults; equal incidence in men and women. Predisposing factors: pregnancy, IBD, immunosuppression.

CLINICAL FEATURES   Presents with severe anal pain + fresh rectal bleeding following defaecation +/– pruritus. 'Sentinel' skin tag/papilla occasionally seen. DRE is usually precluded due to pain.

MANAGEMENT   Approximately 90% settle with conservative measures, i.e. high fibre diet, bulk laxatives, GTN ointment. Failing this, topical calcium channel blockers, botulinum toxin A (Botox) injection or surgery, i.e. lateral sphincterotomy may be beneficial.

Haemorrhoids
Dilated submucosal vascular (haemorrhoidal) cushions within the anal canal. Common in developed countries; equal incidence amongst males and females; peak prevalence 45–65 years. Predisposing factors: straining (e.g. constipation) and obstruction to venous return (e.g. pregnancy).

Classification of haemorrhoids
External (arise below the dentate line) – may be painful
Internal (arise above the dentate line) – can be further classified as:
- **First degree:** Bleed on defaecation but do not prolapse
- **Second degree:** Prolapse with defaecation but reduce spontaneously
- **Third degree:** Prolapse with defaecation requiring manual reduction
- **Fourth degree:** Irreducible

CLINICAL FEATURES
- Bright red, painless rectal bleeding (on toilet paper or in bowel).
- Associated pruritis, prolapse (i.e. mass) and mucus discharge.
- Severe anal pain suggests strangulation or thrombosis.
- Examine for skin tags, thrombosed or prolapsed piles.

INVESTIGATIONS   Proctoscopy: haemorrhoidal cushions typically seen in 3, 7 and 11 o'clock position; exclude malignancy and IBD with flexible sigmoidoscopy, colonoscopy or barium enema.

MANAGEMENT
- Conservative: improve anal hygiene; high fibre diet; bulk laxatives; increase fluid intake and advise avoidance of straining.
- Medical: topical steroids, anaesthetics, antiseptics.
- Surgical: rubber band ligation, injection sclerotherapy (5% phenol in arachis oil); infrared coagulation; cryotherapy or haemorrhoidectomy.
- Thrombosed piles should be managed with bed rest, ice, analgesia +/– topical GTN.

13.15. Abdominal x-ray (AXR)
Systematic analysis of x-rays
The basics
- **Type of x-ray:** i.e. plain abdominal, contrast.
- **Patient details:** name (ethnic origin); hospital number; date of birth, gender.
- **Date of image**.
- **Projection:** PA, AP or lateral.
- **Patient position:** erect versus supine.
- **Adequacy – rotation/penetration:** the vertebral bodies should be clearly visible.

The bowel
- **Intraluminal gas pattern (?normal):** it is usual to see small volumes of gas throughout the GI tract.
- **Look for dilatation of the bowel:** In bowel obstruction, bowel proximal to the obstruction dilates, while the more distal bowel collapses. Normal upper limit for small bowel diameter is 3 cm; large bowel – 6 cm, and caecum – 9 cm. Large and small bowel may be distinguished by looking at the bowel wall markings.
  - Small bowel tends to be central; bowel markings (valvulae conniventes) cross the full diameter of the bowel. Multiple dilated loops of small bowel located centrally within the abdomen plus absence of gas in the large bowel, suggests small bowel obstruction.
  - Large bowel tends to be peripheral; bowel markings (haustra) do not cross full diameter of the bowel.

Other observations
- **Assess soft tissues:** poorly visualised on plain x-ray; however, the kidneys, spleen, liver, bladder (if filled) and psoas muscle shadows can usually be identified.
- **Assess for foreign bodies:** this represents an interesting final observation. Objects seen include those ingested (e.g. batteries); rectal foreign bodies; items in the path of the x-ray beam (e.g. belt buckles); and those deliberately placed, i.e. aortic stents, intra-uterine devices.

  Finally, summarise your key findings.

14

Vascular surgery

14.1. Acute lower limb ischaemia

This is a vascular emergency which if left untreated ('six hour rule') will result in irreversible tissue damage requiring amputation. Classic presentation = 6Ps – Pain, Pallor, Perishing coldness, Pulselessness, Paraesthesia and Paralysis.

Key features in the history
- Symptoms occur acutely.
- Pain is usually sudden in onset, continuous and severe (due to vasospasm); and some relief may be gained by hanging the affected leg from the bed, i.e. dependent blood flow.
- A past history of peripheral vascular disease (PVD), i.e. intermittent claudication, rest pain, ulcers or gangrene suggests an acute on chronic aetiology.
- Risk factors for PVD may be present: diabetes, hypertension, hypercholesterolaemia, smoking, IHD, cerebro- and reno-vascular disease or positive family history.
- Look for evidence suggestive of an embolus, i.e. chest pain, palpitations.

Aetiology of acute lower limb ischaemia

Thrombosis (≈ 60%)
○ Occlusive atherosclerotic disease
○ Graft stenosis
○ Aneurysmal disease: e.g. popliteal aneurysm
○ Coagulopathy/thrombophilia

Embolus (≈ 30%)
○ Atrial fibrillation
○ Mural cardiac thrombus: e.g. post-MI, cardiomyopathy
○ Infective endocarditis, rheumatic heart disease, prosthetic heart valves

○ Thrombus from aneurysmal disease: e.g. AAA, popliteal
○ Atheroma/cholesterol emboli
○ Tumour: e.g. atrial myxoma

Trauma
○ Fracture, joint dislocation
○ Iatrogenic: e.g. arterial cannulation, intra-arterial drug administration

CLINICAL EXAMINATION
- Coldness and pallor.
- Sluggish capillary refill time (>2 secs).
- Absent distal pulses.
- The limb may appear marble white (due to vasospasm).
- As ischaemia progresses, mottling occurs due to vasodilation and stasis of stagnant deoxygenated blood.
- Sensori-motor dysfunction, calf tenderness and a bulging anterior compartment, indicative of muscle necrosis, and fixed mottling are late signs.
- *Note*: weak or absent pulse in the contralateral limb suggests a thrombosis.

INVESTIGATIONS
- Blood tests: FBC (for infection), U&Es (for acute renal failure), CK (for rhabdomyolysis – occurs with muscle breakdown; MI), clotting, thrombophilia screen.
- ABG (metabolic acidosis, lactate – marker of ischaemia).
- Urinalysis: myoglobinuria (suggests rhabdomyolysis).
- ECG: ischaemic changes, MI, AF.
- Imaging: arterial duplex (accurate, non-invasive, useful first-line test); angiography remains the gold standard investigation; CT angiogram scan is indicated if an AAA or aortic dissection is suspected.
- Echocardiogram to exclude a cardiac source of embolism.
- Future management: 24 hour HOLTER monitoring to exclude an arrhythmia.

MANAGEMENT
- Fluid resuscitation + urinary catheterisation and accurate fluid balance assessment.
- IV heparin to prevent further thrombus propagation.
- Opiate analgesia +/– antibiotics.
- Treatment.
  - If limb clinically viable and arterial embolus suspected, embolectomy +/– completion angiogram.
  - If limb viable and thrombosis suspected, angiography, intra-arterial thrombolysis (streptokinase or tPA; takes 4–24 hours to dissolve thrombus), angioplasty, balloon catheter thrombectomy, reconstructive surgery +/– fasciotomies (for compartment syndrome), are possible therapeutic options.
- Post-op: monitor for reperfusion injury and compartment syndrome.
  - If ischaemia is irreversible and the limb non-salvageable, amputation may be required.
  - In select cases, palliative care may be the most appropriate course of action.

14.2. Chronic lower limb ischaemia
Chronic limb ischaemia embraces a spectrum of disease ranging from *intermittent claudication* (a cramp-like pain bought on by walking and relieved with rest) and *rest pain* (pain in the forefoot, typically worse at night, often waking the patient from

their sleep and relieved by hanging the foot over the edge of the bed) to *ulceration* and *gangrene* (irreversible tissue necrosis).

Aetiology: atherosclerosis is commonly implicated and the extent and location of the lesion often correlates with the symptoms, i.e. patients with aorto-iliac disease classically present with buttock claudication and impotence (Leriche's syndrome) those with ilio-femoral disease, thigh claudication and those with femoro-popliteal disease, calf claudication.

Causes of chronic lower limb ischaemia
- ○ Occlusive atherosclerotic disease
- ○ **Vasculitides:** e.g. Buerger's disease; giant-cell arteritis; Takayasu's disease; SLE
- ○ Popliteal entrapment syndrome
- ○ Cystic adventitial disease
- ○ Haematological Disorders
- ○ **Collagen Disorders:** Ehlers-Danlos syndrome and Marfan's syndrome predispose to popliteal aneurysms

Important differential diagnoses
- ○ **Neurological:** spinal canal stenosis (neurogenic claudication)
- ○ **Musculoskeletal:** osteoarthritis
- ○ **Vascular:** venous claudication in a post-phlebitic limb

Critical limb ischaemia
Intermittent claudication affects 5% of men and 2–4% of women over the age of 40 years. Approximately 20% of patients with intermittent claudication will progress to develop critical limb ischaemia where the viability of the limb is threatened.

Critical limb ischaemia as defined by the European Working Group is the presence of ischaemic rest pain requiring analgesia for more than two weeks, or ulceration, or gangrene of the lower extremity with an absolute ankle systolic blood pressure of <50 mmHg and/or toe systolic pressure of <30 mmHg.

CLINICAL EXAMINATION
- Stigmata of vascular disease: e.g. nicotine staining, xanthoma, xanthelasma.
- Cold peripheries, marbled skin, trophic changes (e.g. hairloss and muscle wasting), venous guttering due to a poor inflow.
- Arterial ulcers (usually found over the lateral malleolus), gangrene and previous amputations.
- Capillary refill time >2 seconds.
- Weak/absent distal pulses.
- Buerger's angle (the angle to which the straightened leg must be raised before it turns white) <20° suggests severe ischaemia. *Note:* a normal person can raise their leg to 90° and it will still remain pink.
- A positive Buerger's test, i.e. reactive hyperaemia on hanging the foot to the ground following assessment of Buerger's angle.

INVESTIGATIONS
- Ankle Brachial Pressure Indices (ABPIs). An ABPI of >1.0 is normal. (*Note:* readings can be falsely elevated in diabetic patients due to incompressible calcified vessels.) An ABPI between 0.8 and 0.6 is associated with intermittent claudication and a ratio <0.5 is seen in critical limb ischaemia.
- Imaging: consider arterial duplex, CT angiography or MR angiography; contrast angiography remains the gold-standard (indicated only if intervention is planned).

MANAGEMENT OF CHRONIC LIMB ISCHAEMIA
- Conservative: optimise risk factors:
  - 'stop smoking, keep walking'
  - lifestyle and vascular risk factor management
  - anti-platelet therapy (aspirin 75 mg daily).

  At five years, a third of claudicants with conservative treatment will have improved symptoms; a third will remain stable and a third will progress to critical limb ischaemia.
- Surgical: debilitating claudication may be managed with angioplasty or surgery. However, it should be noted that the mortality within this group at three years is 25% – largely as a result of myocardial infarction or stroke, and fitness for surgery therefore greatly influences management.

MANAGEMENT OF CRITICAL LIMB ISCHAEMIA
- Revascularisation with angioplasty, surgical endarterectomy and/or a bypass procedure is required to salvage the limb.
- Where revascularisation is not possible amputation, lumbar sympathectomy and prostanoids may form part of the management.

14.3. Aneurysms
An aneurysm is a permanent and localised dilatation of a blood vessel to greater than twice its normal diameter. Aneurysms can be classified as:
- true (involving all three layers of the arterial wall) or false (pseudoaneurysms), where partial disruption of the vessel wall results in a contained bleed from the true lumen (usually iatrogenic or traumatic).
- according to their aetiology or shape, i.e. saccular or fusiform.

Aneurysms can occur at any number of sites including the femoral, popliteal, subclavian and carotid arteries. However, the abdominal aorta is the most commonly affected artery (90%).

Aetiology of aneurysms

Congenital: i.e. berry aneurysm affecting arteries of the Circle of Willis in the brain.

Acquired:
- ○ Degenerative (80%)
- ○ Collagen: e.g. Marfan's syndrome; Ehlers-Danlos syndrome, pseudoxanthoma elasticum
- ○ Cystic medial necrosis
- ○ Inflammatory (typically present with back pain, weight loss and raised ESR)
- ○ Infection: mycotic, bacterial (i.e. syphilis), fungal (rare)

Abdominal aortic aneurysms (AAA)
More common in older men and those with a positive family history. Risk factors include smoking, hypertension, hyperlipidaemia and history of PVD. ≈ 95% of all AAAs affect the infra-renal aorta.

CLINICAL FEATURES
- Asymptomatic: diagnosis is incidental in 75%.
- Symptomatic:
  - rupture: symptoms include shock, abdominal/back pain, abdominal distension; exclude in the elderly patient presenting with unexplained hypotension
  - distal ischaemia due to thrombosis or distal embolisation

» epigastric +/– back pain (due to rapid expansion)
» malaise and weight loss (common with inflammatory aneurysms)
» per-rectal bleeding (due to aorto-enteric fistula)
» aortocaval fistula and mass effects.

EXAMINATION
● Pulsatile, expansile, epigastric mass +/– tenderness.
● Shock: confusion, tachycardia, hypotension and oliguria, with rupture.

MANAGEMENT   Depends on whether AAA is symptomatic or asymptomatic

Indications for surgery

○ AAA rupture (surgical emergency) – unless moribund or history of carcinomatosis
○ Symptomatic AAA: increased risk of rupture; symptoms likely related to rapid increase in size
○ Asymptomatic AAA >5.5 cm (risk of rupture 10% per year versus 1% if <4.0 cm) or growth rate of >1 cm per year

Management of ruptured AAA – a surgical emergency
● ABC – insert two large-bore cannulae, perform hypotensive resuscitation, i.e. resuscitation to keep BP below normotension while maintaining the minimum perfusion pressure to adequately perfuse the vital organs (higher BPs cause further blood leak from the AAA), catheterise.
● Send urgent bloods for: FBC, U&Es, clotting, ABG and cross-match eight units blood, FFP and platelets (most units will have an established 'Ruptured AAA Protocol').
● Urgent vascular referral for open/endovascular surgical repair in the fit patient.

Management of an asymptomatic AAA
● Conservative:
  » optimise risk factors: i.e. smoking cessation, low dose aspirin + statin therapy
  » regular follow-up and ultrasound surveillance.
● Surgical:
  » elective surgical repair can be performed via an open or endovascular approach (determined by AAA morphology)
  » work-up for intervention requires assessment of AAA size and morphology, cardiovascular (i.e. echo, ECG, CXR), respiratory (ABG, lung function tests), renal function and includes baseline blood tests (FBC, clotting, U&Es and LFTs).

Complications of open AAA repair

○ Graft kinking, graft thrombosis, distal embolisation, ischaemic bowel
○ Operative mortality of ruptured AAA is 50–70% and for elective repair 2–5%

Screening for AAA
Currently, screening only occurs for high-risk groups, i.e. if family history.

Popliteal aneurysms

Frequently bilateral. ≈ 25% of patients will also have an AAA. Complications include distal embolisation, thrombosis with acute lower limb ischaemia, and rarely rupture.

Visceral aneurysms

Uncommon and usually asymptomatic. Presentation is often with rupture. May affect the hepatic, splenic (classically occurs in pregnancy) and renal arteries. Consider polyarteritis nodosa.

14.4. Ulcers

A break in continuity of an epithelial surface; can be classified by duration – acute or chronic (present for >6 weeks) – or according to the aetiology.

Aetiology of ulcers

- ○ **Vascular:** venous – accounts for 50–75% of all leg ulcers; remainder are arterial or mixed arterial/venous
- ○ **Neuropathic:** commonly associated with diabetes; may be complicated with ischaemia
- ○ **Malignant,** e.g. BCC, SCC, melanoma; accounts for ≈ 2% of all ulcers
- ○ **Vasculitic:** associated with RA and scleroderma
- ○ **Infective,** e.g. TB
- ○ **Trauma, radiation:** e.g. pre-tibial lacerations
- ○ **Pyoderma gangrenosum:** associated with IBD, myeloma, RA and liver disease

EXAMINATION

- Venous ulcers: overly medial aspect of the lower leg; shallow sloping edges with granulation tissue or slough (if infected) at the base; surrounding skin may exhibit evidence of venous disease, e.g. eczema, lipodermatosclerosis.
- Arterial ulcers: overly lateral malleolus, punched out appearance; typically painful; peripheral pulses are usually reduced/absent; patients usually give a history of claudication/rest pain; ABPIs and arterial duplex are useful diagnostic tests.
- Neuropathic ulcers: located in pressure areas, i.e. heel, metatarsal heads; typically deep and painless.
- Malignant ulcers: classically a rolled (basal cell carcinoma (BCC)), or everted edge (squamous cell carcinoma (SCC)); can occur within an existing ulcer, e.g. Marjolin's ulcer. A punch biopsy should be performed if suspected.

MANAGEMENT

- Diabetes mellitus, steroid use, malnutrition, anaemia and oedema all contribute to ulcer formation and healing and should be corrected or optimised. Patient education is key.
- Wound care: regular dressing +/– debridement, wound swabs and antibiotics for infection, serial photographs/ulcer tracing for future comparison.
- Specific treatment:
  - ‣ arterial or mixed venous/arterial ulcers: *see chronic lower limb ischaemia* above
  - ‣ venous ulcers:
    - □ non-surgical management – rest and elevation of the leg, four layer compression bandaging only if ABPI >0.8
    - □ surgical treatment – skin grafting and treatment of primary varicose veins may be beneficial.
  - ‣ Diabetic ulcers: avoid mechanical stress to the limb. A multi-disciplinary approach with referral to a diabetologist, vascular surgeon, podiatrist, is essential.

14.5. Gangrene

Tissue necrosis with putrefaction or mummification. Can be classified as **dry** or **wet**. Dry gangrene is typically well demarcated and will usually auto/self-amputate. Wet gangrene often occurs as a consequence of trauma, acute ischaemia or infection, is poorly demarcated and at risk of spreading.

Causes of gangrene

- ○ Vascular (thrombosis, embolus, critical limb ischaemia, Buerger's disease, Raynaud's disease)
- ○ Diabetes
- ○ Trauma – cold, heat, pressure
- ○ Drug induced: e.g. ergot poisoning

14.6. Amputations

An amputation is indicated if a limb is **dead, dying, or dangerous**.

The most common indication is for lower limb ischaemia. Other indications for surgery include: infection (e.g. gas gangrene, osteomyelitis); trauma; soft tissue/bony malignancy. The level of amputation (e.g. above- or below-knee) is determined by the extent of disease, availability of soft tissue coverage and blood supply of the limb. In general, the more distal the amputation site, the better the functional result, in terms of rehabilitation.

Complications of amputation

Complications may be general or specific to the operation.
- ○ **Immediate:** pain, bleeding + haematoma, psycho-social
- ○ **Early:** phantom limb pain, wound infection and dehiscence, skin necrosis
- ○ **Late:** stump neuroma, osteomyelitis, fixed flexion deformity, rehabilitation problems

MANAGEMENT Involves a multi-disciplinary approach, involving a vascular surgeon, occupational therapist, physiotherapist, rehabilitation physician and prosthetist.

14.7. Vasospastic and sympathetic disorders
Raynaud's phenomenon (RP)

A vasospastic disorder characterised by episodes of digital blanching, followed by cyanosis and rubor (i.e. white to blue to red) typically precipitated by cold or emotion. RP affects 10% of the population to varying degrees and is more common in young women. The aetiology can be classified as: primary (idiopathic) (aka Raynaud's disease) or secondary to another condition (aka Raynaud's syndrome).

CLINICAL FEATURES In addition to colour changes, RP is often associated with parasthesia and occasionally, digital ulceration and gangrene. Other less commonly affected areas are the nose, ears and tongue.

Causes of Raynaud's syndrome

- ○ **Connective tissue diseases (CTD):** scleroderma, SLE, RA, mixed CTD, Sjögren's disease
- ○ **Arterial disease:** Buerger's disease, thoracic outlet syndrome, embolism, atherosclerosis
- ○ **Occupational:** vibrating tools
- ○ **Trauma:** frostbite, trench foot

○ **Blood dyscrasias:** cold agglutinins, cryoglobinaemia, myeloproliferative disease
○ **Drugs:** β-blockers, oestrogens, nicotine, bleomycin, ergotamine, bromocriptine, sulphasalazine
○ **Endocrine:** hypothyroidism, carcinoid syndrome

INVESTIGATIONS – DIRECTED TOWARDS IDENTIFYING A TREATABLE CAUSE
- Blood tests: ESR, TFTs, ANA, RF, blood glucose, serum protein electrophoresis, cryoglobulins.
- CXR for fibrosis in CTD and cervical rib.
- Arterial duplex +/– angiography.
- Capillary nailfold microscopy (diagnostic for RP).

MANAGEMENT
- Patient education with avoidance of precipitating factors, i.e. cold, cessation of smoking and biofeedback.
- If conservative treatment fails, calcium channel antagonists/α-blockers which act as vasodilators, may prove beneficial.
- Other potentially useful medications: iloprost (synthetic prostacyclin agonist).
- In severe disease, consider upper thoracic sympathectomy.

Hyperhidrosis
Abnormal excessive sweating due to sympathetic overactivity. Affects 1% of the population and may be generalised or focal – commonly affecting the axillae, palms of the hands, soles of the feet or forehead. Often very socially embarrassing for the patient.

Can be classified as primary (idiopathic) hyperhidrosis or secondary to hyperthyroidism, phaechromocytoma, obesity, drugs, e.g. glucocorticosteroids, antidepressants, stress, and anxiety. Management: topical antiperspirants, anticholinergics and botulinum toxin A; with surgery reserved for resistant cases, i.e. thoracoscopic/lumbar sympathectomy.

14.8. Varicose veins
Dilated, tortuous and elongated superficial veins. Commonly affects the long saphenous vein (LSV) ($\approx 90\%$) due to incompetence at the saphenofemoral junction (SFJ); the short saphenous vein (SSV) due to incompetence at the saphenopopliteal junction (SPJ) and rarely in isolation, the calf perforator veins. More common in women, often presenting after pregnancy.

Aetiology of varicose

Primary: due to congenitally absent or abnormal valves

Secondary:
○ Problems affecting the valves (thrombosis, thrombophlebitis)
○ Problems affecting the muscle pump (immobility, stroke, joint stiffness)
○ Factors affecting venous return (DVT, pregnancy, ascites, obesity, pelvic/abdominal mass)

HISTORY
- Aching, pruritis, cramps, heaviness and swelling of the legs often after periods of standing (ask about occupation, i.e. teacher, shop assistant).
- Skin changes, ulcers, and symptoms of superficial thrombophlebitis.
- Past medical history of deep vein thrombosis (DVT).

EXAMINATION

- Spider veins, prominent varicosities, sapheno-varix, venous eczema, hyperpigmentation, lipodermatosclerosis (thickening and hardening of the skin and subcutaneous tissues), ulcers (classically, overlying the medial malleolus in the gaitor region).
- Positive cough impulse due to SFJ or SPJ incompetence.
- Specific tests:
  - tap test.
  - Trendelenberg test/tourniquet test – useful for assessing level of reflux along the LSV
  - Perthes test (often talked about, rarely performed) – used to exclude deep venous incompetence
  - hand held doppler – valuable for demonstrating SFJ or SPJ incompetence.
- Investigations: venous duplex (for complex or recurrent varicose veins).

MANAGEMENT

- Conservative.
  - Graduated compression hosiery (exclude arterial disease before use). Weight loss, regular exercise, elevate legs and avoidance of prolonged periods of standing.
- Surgical (indicated for venous ulceration or symptomatic varicose veins).
  - High tie and stripping of the LSV and multiple avulsions under GA. Complications: bleeding, groin infection, thrombophlebitis, DVT, damage to the saphenous nerve and recurrence.
  - Newer therapies: endovenous ultrasound (VNUS Closure) or endovenous laser therapy (EVLT) and foam sclerotherapy; performed under LA.

14.9. Deep vein thrombosis (DVT)

DVT is a thrombosis occurring within the deep venous system of the lower limb. (They occur less commonly in the subclavian, visceral veins and vena cava). Clinical features: commonly unilateral swelling, pain and redness of the calf.

Complications: pulmonary embolus (PE), post-phlebitic syndrome (recanalisation but with loss of valve function leading to symptoms of chronic venous insufficiency, i.e. pigmentation, lipodermatosclerosis and ulceration) and failure of recanalisation leading to persistence of symptoms of venous obstruction, i.e. swelling, pain on exercising (venous claudication).

Risk factors for DVT

Patient factors

- Age >40 years
- Pregnancy
- OCP or HRT
- Female gender
- Obesity
- Previous DVT/PE
- Prothrombotic tendency: inherited thrombophilias, protein C, protein S and antithrombin deficiencies and genetic mutations, i.e. factor V Leiden and prothrombin 20210A variant

Operative/pathological factors

- Major abdominal or pelvic surgery
- Surgery duration >150 mins
- Sepsis
- Malignancy
- Laparoscopic procedure
- Post-operative immobility >4 days
- Pelvic or long bone fracture
- Congestive cardiac failure

INVESTIGATIONS

- D-Dimer (a fibrin degradation product): highly sensitive for thrombosis (>90%), but has low specificity (30–40%).
- Venous duplex scanning of the deep system; first-line, non-invasive test.
- Thrombophilia screen.
- Abdominal/pelvic ultrasound or CT (to exclude malignancy).

MANAGEMENT   Patient should be treated on the suspicion of a DVT. Treatment is aimed at preventing clot propagation thus minimising the risk of PE and facilitating resolution of the thrombus. Options:
- anticoagulation with initially heparin followed by warfarin for 3–6 months
- thrombolysis: indicated in cases of massive PE
- inferior vena caval filter insertion: e.g. if anticoagulation is contra-indicated.

DVT preventative strategies

- ○ **Pre-operatively:** e.g. weight loss TEDS (graduated compression stockings), subcutaneous Heparin injections (continue till mobile post-operatively)
- ○ **Intra-operatively:** e.g. ankle rests (to elevate calves), TEDS
- ○ **Post-operatively:** e.g. early mobilisation, TEDS and heparin

14.10. Lymphoedema

An accumulation of protein rich fluid in the interstitium due to an abnormality of the lymphatic system.

Aetiology of lymphoedema

- ○ **Primary:** cause is unclear; may be congenital; if familial termed Milroy's disease
- ○ **Secondary:** more common; surgical excision of lymph nodes, radiotherapy, infections (*Wuchereria bancrofti, mycobacterium tuberculosis*), malignant infiltration of lymphatics

CLINICAL FEATURES

- Commonly, affects the legs (≈ 90% of cases), less frequently arms, genitalia and face.
- Usually unilateral and pitting in the early stages.
- Swelling typically increases throughout the day and is worse on standing.
- Associated with an increased risk of superficial skin infections.

INVESTIGATIONS

- Diagnosis is clinical following exclusion of other causes of limb swelling.
- Where the diagnosis is unclear, isotope or contrast lymphangiography, lymphoscintography may be useful.

Other causes of a swollen limb

- ○ Systemic causes: heart failure, hypoproteinaemia, renal failure, hepatic failure
- ○ Venous causes: post-phlebitic limb, iliac vein occlusion
- ○ Extrinsic pressure: pelvic/abdominal masses, ascites
- ○ Other: obesity, limb disuse, arteriovenous malformation, allergies, angio-oedema

MANAGEMENT

- Conservative: compression stockings, external pneumatic compression, elevate limb, supportive therapy (e.g. foot and skin care to minimise risk of infection), aggressive management of infections.

- Surgical: Debulking procedures, bypass operations and liposuction.

15

Urology

15.1. Haematuria

Blood in the urine can be categorised as *macroscopic* (frank) or *microscopic* (found incidentally on urine dipstick or microscopy), or as *painful* or *painless*.

All patients with a persistent macroscopic haematuria or microscopic/dipstick haematuria of >3 months duration require investigation.

Causes of haematuria

○ Renal tract stones: ureteric stones, bladder stones
○ Prostate disease: benign prostatic hypertrophy
○ Tumours: e.g. adeno-, transitional or squamous cell carcinoma of the kidneys, ureter or bladder
○ Infection: bacterial, mycobacterial (e.g. TB), parasitic (e.g. schistosomiasis)
○ Polycystic kidney disease: bleeding cyst
○ Immune-mediated: e.g. IgA nephropathy, glomerulonephritis, vasculitis
○ Bleeding dyscrasias: congenital, e.g. haemophilia; acquired, e.g. anticoagulation therapy
○ Vascular: e.g. renal infarction secondary to embolus (consider if patient is in AF)
○ Trauma

INVESTIGATIONS

● Confirm the presence of blood in urine with microscopy, and exclude infection with urine MC&S. Send urine for cytology.
● Blood tests: FBC, U&Es, CRP and clotting.
● Image the renal tract: ultrasound, KUB (for calculi); IVU or more commonly CT KUB; retrograde ureterography in select cases and staging CT (if malignancy suspected).
● Flexible cystoscopy +/− biopsy.

MANAGEMENT
- ABC, correct clotting and transfuse as necessary.
- Treat underlying cause.
- If risk of clot retention from heavy blood loss, catheterise using a three-way Foley catheter and irrigate the bladder.

15.2. Lower urinary tract symptoms (LUTS)

Most commonly due to benign prostatic hyperplasia, infection, inflammation or neoplasia of the prostate, urethra or pelvic organs. Other causes include: bladder outflow obstruction (BOO) and cauda equina syndrome. Clinical features (*see* below).

Symptoms related to difficulty in voiding

- Hesitancy
- Intermittent flow
- Straining
- Sensation of incomplete emptying
- Poor stream
- Dysuria
- Post-micturition dribbling
- Nocturia

Symptoms related to difficulty in storing urine

- Frequency
- Urgency

INVESTIGATIONS
- Urine MC&S/MSU.
- FBC, U&Es, PSA.
- Imaging: renal tract ultrasound (for hydronephrosis, or malignancy), transrectal ultrasound biopsy (TRUS) (if prostate suspicious on digital rectal examination), flexible cystoscopy (to exclude urethral and bladder pathology).

MANAGEMENT   Depends on the underlying cause.

Urinary retention

This is an inability to empty the bladder and may arise due to a mechanical obstruction or reduced detrusor power. Urinary retention can be classified according to duration as *acute* or *chronic*.

Acute retention
- Normally painful
- Causes: prostatic enlargement, urinary tract infection, constipation, pain, drugs (e.g. anticholinergics, alpha-agonists), GA, alcohol, infection
- Clinical features: patients typically present with a history of not passing urine, suprapubic pain and tenderness +/– a palpable bladder
- Management: catheterise promptly to relieve pain. An underlying cause should be sought and treated accordingly

Chronic retention
- Normally painless. The bladder capacity is usually increased to >1.5 litres and there may also be overflow incontinence
- Causes: prostatic enlargement, drugs (e.g. antidepressants), pelvic malignancy, neurological disease (e.g. multiple sclerosis, Parkinson's disease)
- Clinical features: on examination there is a palpable, non-tender bladder and there may be evidence of renal failure (US for hydronephrosis)
- Management: catheterise; look for an underlying cause and treat

15.3. Benign prostatic hyperplasia (BPH)

Common, affecting half of all men over the age of 45. In many men over the age of 60, symptoms become unacceptable and require treatment.

CLINICAL FEATURES
- LUTS.
- Difficulty passing urine (+/– urinary retention).
- Haematuria.
- DRE: enlarged +/– tender prostate gland.
- Complications if untreated include recurrent UTIs, bladder diverticulum, bladder calculi due to stagnant urine, renal failure in chronic retention.

INVESTIGATIONS
- Blood tests: FBC, U&Es (for renal failure), PSA (do not perform immediately following DRE or catheterisation as result may be falsely elevated).
- Urinalysis (for haematuria and infection), urine MC&S.
- Post-voiding residual volume – should be 0 ml, i.e.patients should normally be able to completely empty their bladder.
- Flow rate studies, i.e. for assessment of urine flow against time.
- Pressure flow studies to investigate renal tract obstruction.
- Renal tract ultrasound: for hydronephrosis.
- TRUS (Transrectal Ultrasound) + biopsy – if PSA elevated.

MANAGEMENT
- Urethral catheter if in retention.
- Medical:
  - alpha-blockers: e.g. tamsulosin – relaxes the bladder neck
  - 5-alpha reductase inhibitors: e.g. finasteride – inhibits the conversion of testosterone to dihydrotesterone
  - anticholinergics: e.g. oxybutynin – reduces symptoms of frequency and urgency
- Surgery – indicated if symptoms are severe, failed medical therapy; recurrent UTIs or renal failure (chronic retention and renal failure require urinary catheter insertion while awaiting surgery). Options:
  - transurethral resection of prostate (TURP)
  - newer procedures: e.g. transurethral radiofrequency needle ablation (TUNA) and laser prostatectomy
  - open/radical prostatectomy: if prostate large or recurrence.

TUR syndrome

This is a well-recognised complication of TURP and is due to excessive glycine reabsorption causing dilutional hyponatraemia. Clinical features: hypotension, bradycardia and confusion. Management: exclude post-operative shock as a cause (e.g. septicaemia or haemorrhage), correct electrolyte imbalance, fluid restrict. Avoid in future procedures, by using normal saline as an irrigation fluid.

15.4. Urinary tract infection (UTI)

The presence of a pure growth of colony forming units within the urinary tract, which leads to an inflammatory response by the urothelium. Symptoms depend on the site of the infection, which may occur within the bladder (cystitis), prostate (prostatitis) or kidneys (pyelonephritis). The most commonly implicated organisms are Gram-negative bacteria such as *E. coli*, *Klebsiella* and *Proteus*.

UTIs may be *complicated* or *uncomplicated*.
- *Complicated UTIs:* occur in the presence of underlying anatomical or functional abnormalities, e.g. renal tract stones, and can be difficult to manage.
- *Uncomplicated UTIs:* occur in the absence of any underlying structural abnormality; they commonly occur in women and respond well to antibiotic treatment.

CLINICAL FEATURES
- Cystitis: frequency, small volume voids, suprapubic pain, urgency, cloudy urine, haematuria and urethral burning on voiding (dysuria).
- Pyelonephritis: fever and rigors, malaise, loin pain, frequency, urgency, dysuria.

INVESTIGATIONS
- Most uncomplicated UTIs will not need investigation beyond urinalysis (positive nitrites and leucocytes); send sample sent for MC&S.
- However if unwell, FBC, U&Es, CRP, blood cultures should be be performed.
- Imaging of the renal tract (ultrasound +/– CT KUB) is indicated to investigate recurrent UTIs when a structural cause is suspected.

MANAGEMENT
- Cystitis: oral antibiotics, e.g. trimethoprim, nitrofurantoin or cefalexin.
- Acute pyelonephritis: hospital admission, analgesia + IV antibiotics, e.g. cefuroxime +/– gentamicin until pyrexia resolves.

15.5. Renal cancer
Renal cell carcinoma (RCC)
Most common renal malignancy. Usually sporadic but may occur in association with hereditary diseases such as Von Hippel-Lindau syndrome. Spread can be: direct (into renal vein, inferior vena cava and right atrium); lymphatic (to the para-aortic and hilar lymph nodes) or haematogenous (to the lungs, liver, bone and brain).

CLINICAL FEATURES
- Haematuria, loin pain + renal mass.
- Night sweats, fever, fatigue.
- Palpable renal-angle mass +/– varicocele.
- Signs of paraneoplastic syndromes: e.g. conjunctival pallor due to anaemia, cushingoid facies, gynaecomastia and baldness.
- Hypercalcaemia due to bone metastases or excess production of PTH-related peptide by the tumour.

INVESTIGATIONS
- Blood tests: FBC (for anaemia or polycythaemia), U&Es (for renal impairment), LFTs (deranged in metastatic disease).
- Urine cytology, microscopy and culture: usually normal.
- Imaging: ultrasound for a renal mass; CXR for cannon ball metastasis; staging CT of the abdomen + chest; MRI – if renal vein involvement.

MANAGEMENT
- Haematuria may require 3-way catheter + irrigation +/– blood transfusion.
- Surgical options include:
  - radical nephrectomy (via an open or laparoscopic approach)

⟩ partial nephrectomy (suitable for multifocal or bilateral tumours) with annual long-term follow-up for recurrence of local disease
⟩ palliative surgery; adjuvant radiotherapy and immunotherapy, arterial embolisation may form part the treatment in advanced cancers.

Transitional cell carcinoma also affects the kidney.

15.6. Bladder cancer
Transitional cell carcinoma (TCC)
Most common bladder malignancy. Can be single or multifocal. Patients often have synchronous upper tract TCC and recurrences are common. TCC is clinically classified as superficial or muscle invasive and can also affect the renal pelvis or ureters. Spread is via direct extension, lymphatics (to para-aortic, para-caval and pelvic nodes), or haematogenous (to liver, lungs and bone).

Risk factors for TCC bladder

○ Male gender
○ Increasing age (>65 years)
○ Smoking
○ Chronic inflammation of bladder mucosa
○ Occupational exposure to aromatic amines such as benzidine and β-naphthylamine

CLINICAL FEATURES
● Painless haematuria: may be initial or terminal depending on whether lesion is at bladder neck or prostatic urethra, respectively; or microscopic haematuria found incidentally on urinalysis.
● Acute retention due to outflow obstruction.
● Lower urinary tract symptoms (e.g. urgency).
● Recurrent UTIs.
● Pneumaturia (due to colovesical fistula).
● Umbilical discharge (with urachal adenocarcinomas).
● Suprapubic mass: suggests locally advanced disease.
● DRE: mass above or involving prostate gland.

INVESTIGATIONS
● Blood tests: FBC (low Hb, high WCC), U&Es.
● Urine dipstick and MC&S; urine cytology.
● Imaging: renal tract ultrasound; CT KUB.
● Flexible cystoscopy.
● Staging investigations: pelvic CT or MRI for extra-vesical tumour extension or iliac lymphadenopathy; CXR for lung metastases; isotope bone scan.

MANAGEMENT Depends on grade of cancer and spread, i.e. whether superficial or muscle invasive.
● Superficial: options include transurethral resection of bladder tumour (TURBT), intravesical chemotherapy (e.g. Mitomycin-C, intravesical BCG).
● Muscle invasive: options include TURBT +/− chemotherapy, palliative radiotherapy, partial cystectomy +/− chemotherapy, radical cystectomy + ileal conduit formation or neobladder formation, ureterosigmoidostomy.
● Metastatic bladder cancer: options include systemic chemotherapy (e.g. using cisplatin, methotrexate and vinblastin) +/− palliative radiotherapy.

Other bladder cancers
- **Squamous cell carcinoma** (associated with chronic inflammation, e.g. bladder calculi or *Schistosomiasis*).
- **Adenocarcinoma** (rare).

15.7. Prostate cancer

Normally adenocarcinoma. Typically occurs in the peripheral zone of the prostate, and often multifocal. Common cancer in men, with a higher incidence in Afro-Caribbeans. Screening now advised between ages 50–70 years, with prostate specific antigen (PSA) assay + digital DRE. Spread can be local, haematogenous and lymphatic to liver, lungs, testis, brain and bone.

CLINICAL FEATURES
- Lower urinary tract symptoms, urinary retention, haematuria (+/– anaemia) and pain due to local spread.
- DRE: large, nodular or fixed, craggy, asymmetrical prostate gland.
- Pathological fractures, spinal cord compression due to bony metastases.

INVESTIGATIONS
- Blood tests: FBC (for anaemia), U&E, LFTs (abnormal in metastatic disease), PSA (not always elevated in high-grade cancers), acid and alkaline phosphatase and serum calcium (high in bony metastases).
- Imaging: renal tract ultrasound; transrectal ultrasound (TRUS) + biopsy for histology; staging CXR (for lung metastasis); CT chest, abdomen and pelvis +/– bone scan (for advanced disease); note sclerotic lesions on plain X-ray.

Gleeson scoring

This is an important prognostic indicator. The gland is microscopically graded 1–5 according to its glandular architecture. The two dominant grades are added to give a score between 2–10. If only one grade is seen the score is doubled:
- ○ 2–4 = well differentiated
- ○ 5–7 = moderately differentiated
- ○ 8–10 = poorly differentiated

MANAGEMENT
- Watchful waiting with six-monthly follow-up, indicated if Gleeson score 2–4; or Gleeson score 5–6 and patient >75 years old.
- If localised, options include:
  - radical prostatectomy +/– radiotherapy or hormone therapy
  - brachytherapy.
- If metastatic, options include:
  - **androgen dependent:** androgen reduction can lead to improvement, e.g. bilateral orchidectomy, LHRH agonists (such as goserelin), bicalutamide (an anti-androgen)
  - **androgen independent:** oestrogens (e.g. diethylstilboesterol), cytotoxic chemotherapy for symptomatic relief
  - **palliation of pain:** analgesia (NSAIDs particularly effective), local radiotherapy, bisphosphonates.

15.8. Penile disorders
Phimosis
Inability to retract foreskin, secondary to narrowing of preputial ring. Aetiology:

although caused by balanitis, phimosis can also predispose to balanitis and is thus a vicious circle.

CLINICAL FEATURES   Poor stream or pain on sexual intercourse.

MANAGEMENT   Surgery is indicated if symptomatic or recurrent balanitis (e.g. circumcision).

Paraphimosis

Inability to pull a retracted foreskin back over the glans penis. This leads to oedema of the glans making it even more difficult to replace the foreskin. It is often painful and typically occurs in hospitals in elderly men following urethral catheterisation. If untreated, it can lead to ischaemia and gangrene of the glans penis.

MANAGEMENT   Give analgesia and attempt manual reduction with topical lignocaine gel (also acts as a lubricant). If this fails, consider surgery, i.e. dorsal slit or circumcision.

Priapism

Persistent (and painful) penile erection without sexual desire. Causes: drugs, malignancy (e.g.leukaemia), sickle cell disease, penile vein thrombosis and spinal cord lesions.

MANAGEMENT   May respond to ice packs but if this fails then drain with needle inserted into corpora and aspirate blood. If a low-flow syndrome then local injection of phenylephrine may help. Surgery is rarely necessary.

Peyronie's disease

An abnormal curvature of the penis due to fibrosis of the tunica albuginea. This is worse when there is an erection and associated with pain, which makes sexual intercourse difficult/impossible. Occurs between 40–60 years of age and is associated with Dupuytren's contracture and HLA-B27 antigen positivity.

MANAGEMENT   May resolve spontaneously but surgical management is occasionally required.

15.9. Testicular disorders

Causes of testicular lumps

- ○ **Within testis:** tumour, orchitis, testicular torsion
- ○ **Separate:** hydrocele, varicocele, epididymal cyst, epididymitis, inguino-scrotal hernia

Testicular tumours

Benign tumours (e.g. Leydig or Sertoli cell tumours) are rare. More commonly tumours are malignant, occurring in 20–40 year old men. Includes: seminomas, teratomas, mixed teratoma-seminomas and lymphomas (in older men).

CLINICAL FEATURES   Painless scrotal lump (often detected by patient or partner) which is hard, irregular/craggy, ill-defined, non-transilluminable and whose upper extent cannot be palpated. Mass may be associated with a reactive hydrocele (rare) or have features of metastatic disease, e.g. SOB.

MANAGEMENT

- Investigations: testicular ultrasound +/– staging CT and refer to a urologist urgently.
- Surgery: radical orchidectomy – excision of testis, epididymis and cord through a groin incision (this incision reduces the risk of lymphatic spread) +/– interval silicone prosthesis insertion.
- Counselling regarding infertility and sperm preservation prior to chemotherapy or radiotherapy – radiotherapy if seminoma, chemotherapy if teratoma.

Varicocele

Varicose veins of the pampiniform plexus. Common (more so on the left) and generally asymptomatic (occasionally a dull ache). Lump often described as a 'bag of worms'; worse on standing. Associated with infertility but cause and effect not clear.

INVESTIGATIONS   Ultrasound of testes and renal tract (to exclude tumour) should be performed.

MANAGEMENT   Treat only if painful or for infertility, with surgical ligation or embolisation.

Hydrocele

Excessive fluid in the tunica vaginalis. May be primary or secondary (due to a reaction to testicular pathology).

CLINICAL FEATURES   Mass is fluctuant, soft (rarely, may be tense), painless and transilluminates.

MANAGEMENT   Treat with aspiration (although high likelihood of recurrence) or surgical excision, and exclude underlying pathology.

Testicular torsion

Typically occurs in children or adolescent males. Testis twists on spermatic cord impeding the blood flow to testis.

CLINICAL FEATURES   Sudden onset of pain within the hemi-scrotum typically radiating to the groin and/or loin with associated nausea and vomiting. May be a history of preceding trauma or bike riding, fever. On examination, there is scrotal swelling + tenderness, a high-riding testis ± hydrocele. Diagnosis is clinical.

MANGEMENT   Treat with analgesia, urgent referral to urologist + surgical exploration/orchidopexy (ideally within 6 hours of onset of symptoms).

Orthopaedics

16.1. Fractures

A fracture is a break in the continuity of a bone associated with a soft tissue injury. They can be categorised in various ways, according to:

- integrity of the overlying skin: **open** (compound) – skin disrupted; **closed** – skin intact
- extent of bone cortex injury: **incomplete** – only one cortex is involved; **complete** – both cortices are involved
- aetiology: i.e. **traumatic, stress** or **pathological**
- pattern of fracture: i.e. **oblique, spiral, transverse, comminuted** (>2 fragments) **impacted** (crush), **displaced** or **undisplaced**.

Note, the nature (direct or indirect) and magnitude of the applied force will determine the fracture pattern, which in turn, will determine its stability, i.e. transverse fractures produced by direct forces are more stable compared to oblique or spiral fractures caused by axial loading and torsional forces, respectively.

Types of fracture

- ○ **Greenstick:** occur in children where the bones are more pliable and tend to bend rather than break, resulting in an *incomplete* fracture
- ○ **Pathological:** occur in bone weakened by disease, e.g. metastases, Paget's disease
- ○ **Stress:** caused by low intensity cyclical loading, e.g. March fracture of the second metatarsal

MANAGEMENT

- ABC with cervical spine immobilisation (as per ATLS™ guidelines).
- Analgesia; assessment of the neurovascular status of the limb.
- Imaging: x-ray all of fractured limb including the joint above and below.
- Open fractures are classified according to the *Gustilo and Anderson*

classification and unlike closed fractures, they carry a risk of contamination and infection. In addition to the above, open fractures require:
- tetanus prophylaxis
- wound swab for MC&S followed by systemic broad spectrum antibiotics
- photography of the wound before covering with betadine/saline soaked gauze
- surgical debridement and wound irrigation within **six hours** of injury; with inspection +/– delayed closure of the wound at 48 hours.
- Reduction of the fracture – achieved either via an open or closed method. Indications for open reduction include: failed closed reduction; an open, unstable, intra-articular or pathological fracture; if neurovascular compromise/ multiple injuries.
- Stabilisation of the fracture – achieved using internal (i.e. plates, k-wires) or external fixation (i.e. rigid cast; skin traction (Thomas' splint) or skeletal traction).
- Immobilisation of the limb to allow healing.
- Rehabilitation + physiotherapy.

Aims of fracture treatment

Fracture reduction: limits soft tissue injury and further bleeding, reduces risk of fat embolisation, relieves pain, restores vascular supply to limb, facilitates transportation.

Fracture fixation: maintains position, allows union without deformity.

Immobilisation: facilitates fracture healing.

Rehabilitation: restores limb function.

Fracture Healing
Bone healing can be either primary or secondary. The latter is the more common.
- **Primary** bony union or fracture healing occurs when there is absolute stability, i.e. no movement between fracture surfaces under a functional load, as seen with rigid internal fixation.
- **Secondary** fracture healing occurs when there is relative stability and has five overlapping phases: 1) tissue destruction and haematoma formation, 2) inflammation and cellular proliferation, 3) callus formation, 4) consolidation and 5) remodelling.

Time scales for fracture healing
- Callus visible: upper limb and lower limb 2 weeks
- Union: upper limb 4–6 weeks, lower limb 8–12 weeks

Factors affecting fracture healing
- **General factors:** age, co-morbidity, nutritional status, alcoholism, drugs such as steroids, smoking, radiation.
- **Local factors:** mobility at fracture site, separation of the bone ends, interruption of the blood supply, type of fracture (displaced and comminuted fractures tend to take longer to heal) and infection.

Complications of fractures

Immediate
- Bleeding +/– haematoma
- Neurovascular injury
- Fat embolus +/– ARDS

Early
○ Compartment syndrome: intrafascial compartment pressures >30–40 mmHg
○ Infection
○ Deep vein thrombosis +/– pulmonary embolus

Late
○ Mal-union: union of the fracture with an angular or rotational deformity or unacceptable shortening
○ Delayed union: an absence of fracture union within the expected time frame, as assessed radiologically
○ Non-union: failure of union
○ Volkmann's ischaemic contracture
○ Joint stiffness, loss/limitation of function and early osteoarthritis
○ Avascular necrosis
○ Myositis ossificans (abnormal calcification within the soft tissue)
○ Growth disturbance (seen if the fracture affects the growth plate in children)
○ Sudeck's atrophy (chronic pain in the affected limb)

16.2. Upper limb disorders
Dislocation of the shoulder
In 95% of cases the glenohumeral joint dislocates anteriorly, in 4% posteriorly and rarely superiorly. (*Dislocation is defined as loss of congruity between the articulating surfaces of a joint.*)

● *Anterior dislocations* typically follow abduction, extension and external rotation injuries, e.g. falls onto an outstretched arm classically in the elderly. They risk damaging the axillary artery and nerve – the latter innervates deltoid and a 'regimental badge' area of skin over the upper lateral aspect of the arm.

● *Posterior dislocations* arise from excessive adduction and internal rotation, e.g. during seizures or following electrocution.

MANAGEMENT   Assess for neurovascular compromise; x-ray (AP + 'Y' views); analgesia; relocate the joint, e.g. using the Hippocratic or Kocher's method and repeat X-ray to confirm successful relocation.

Shoulder pain
Can arise from the joint itself, from the muscles/tendons surrounding the joint or be referred from elsewhere.

Causes
○ Adhesive capsulitis (frozen shoulder)
○ Rotator cuff tear
○ Rotator cuff impingement
○ Calcific tendonitis
○ Degenerative disease: e.g. osteoarthritis

Fractures of the upper limb *(see above for general fracture management)*

Fractures of the clavicle
Mechanism of injury: commonly follows a direct blow over the clavicle or falling on an outstretched hand.

CLINICAL FEATURES   Pain and deformity; the middle third of the clavicle is most frequently affected.

MANAGEMENT   Fractures of the middle third of the clavicle can be managed conservatively with a broad arm sling + rehabilitation; fractures of the distal or proximal clavicle often require open reduction + internal fixation (ORIF).

Fractures of the proximal humerus
May involve the anatomical neck, more commonly the surgical neck or greater and lesser tuberosities of the humerus. Mechanism of injury: typically follows a fall on an outstretched hand, in an elderly patient.

CLINICAL FEATURES   Swelling and bruising of the shoulder girdle, and joint crepitus. *Note*: the brachial plexus, axillary nerve and artery are at risk of damage.

MANAGEMENT   Analgesia; exclude neurovascular compromise; x-ray +/− CT; if fracture is undisplaced treat conservatively; displaced fractures require ORIF.

Fractures of the shaft of the humerus
Mechanism of injury: typically due to direct trauma or a twisting injury (resulting in a spiral fracture). If spontaneous, consider underlying pathology; in children, consider abuse if the purported mechanism is inconsistent with the injury.

CLINICAL FEATURES   Swelling, bruising and pain on elbow or shoulder movement. *Note*: the radial nerve is frequently damaged (look for wrist drop).

MANAGEMENT   Analgesia; x-ray (occasionally CT or MRI) to confirm diagnosis. Treatment includes: plaster casting, humeral brace or ORIF, i.e. intramedullary nailing/plating + rehabilitation.

Supracondylar (distal humeral) fractures of the humerus
Rare in adults, but the most common fracture affecting children. Mechanism of injury: often occurs following a fall on an outstretched hand. *Note*: the brachial artery is at risk of damage.

CLINICAL FEATURES
A swollen, painful elbow held in semi-flexion.

MANAGEMENT   Closed/open reduction with the position maintained with a backslab + collar and cuff is required. Monitor for compartment syndrome.

Fractures of the shaft of the radius and ulna
- **Monteggia injury:** a displaced fracture of the shaft of the ulna, associated with dislocation of the radial head. Due to instability these fractures require ORIF of the ulnar fracture and reduction of the radial head.
- **Galeazzi fracture-dislocation:** a fracture of the radius, associated with a dislocation of the distal radio-ulnar joint. Management is as above.
- **Nightstick fracture:** an isolated, minimally displaced fracture of the ulna – usually in the midshaft. Termed 'nightstick' as historically sustained whilst defending a blow from a nightstick with the forearm.

Fractures of the distal radius – may be intra- or extra-articular
- **Colles' fracture:** extra-articular fracture of the distal radius (within 2.5 cm of the wrist joint) with dorsal angulation and radial shortening resulting in a 'dinner-fork' deformity. Commonly occurs in the elderly following a fall on an

outstretched hand. Management: requires manipulation, usually under regional anaesthesia (e.g. Bier's block), fixation in a below-elbow plaster cast for six weeks, regular follow-up x-rays to check position and rehabilitation. Beware of non-union, median nerve palsy and extensor pollicis longus (EPL) tendon rupture.

- **Smith's fracture:** extra-articular fracture of the distal radius with volar angulation. Management: requires manipulation, fixation in an above-elbow plaster cast for six weeks, regular follow-up x-rays to check position and rehabilitation.
- **Barton's fracture:** intra-articular fracture of the distal radius. Commonly requires ORIF, i.e. with k-wires, plating.

16.3. Lower limb fractures and dislocations

Fractures of the pelvis

Mortality of ≈ 20%; can produce significant haemorrhage (up to 4 L). Four mechanisms identified: anterior-posterior (AP) compression; lateral compression (motor vehicle accidents); vertical shear forces (fall from a height); or a combination. *Note*: the pelvis is a ring-shaped structure; fracture at one point, implies there must be a fracture or dislocation at another point.

CLINICAL FEATURES
- Shock.
- 'Destot sign' (haematoma above the inguinal ligament or upper thigh/scrotum).
- Pelvic tenderness ('springing' or instability on bimanual compression or distraction of the iliac wings).
- Signs of associated injury: urethral (high-riding prostate, blood at the urethral meatus and scrotal haematoma), vaginal, rectal, abdominal, lower limb neurovascular.

MANAGEMENT   According to ATLS™ guidelines with orthopaedic, urology, general surgical and radiological input.
- Resuscitation.
- Image: x-ray (AP +/– oblique pelvic views); CT (if haemodynamically stable); consider FAST (Focused Assessment with Sonography for Trauma) ultrasound (for pelvic blood), urethrography (if urethral injury suspected) and angiography +/– embolisation.
- Stabilise the pelvis, e.g. with a circumferentially placed sheet, external fixator or C-clamp, to tamponade bleeding.
- Treat associated injuries: e.g. urethral, as appropriate.

Dislocation of the hip

Commonly associated with trauma; ≈ 10% will also have a pelvic fracture. Can be classified as anterior, posterior or central. Posterior dislocations are more common and occur due to a posterior force applied on a flexed knee and hip, e.g. when the knee strikes the dashboard in a head-on collision. Management includes resuscitation, analgesia, AP + lateral hip x-rays with early relocation to reduce the risk of avascular necrosis (AVN) of the femoral head.

Fractures of the neck of femur (#NOF)

Common in the elderly (mean age 80 years; 3:1 male to female ratio); frequently occurs following a simple fall; associated with a 20–40% mortality at one year. Clinical features: the leg is shortened and externally rotated and the patient is usually unable to weight-bear due to pain. Can be classified as intracapsular or extracapsular.

- **Extracapsular fractures:** are subdivided as basi-cervical, intertrochanteric and subtrochanteric. Unlike intracapsular fractures, they are not associated with a significant risk of AVN. Management: can be conservatively with traction or more commonly, surgically with internal fixation, i.e. cannulated screws.
- **Intracapsular fractures:** are subdivided as subcapital and transcervical; and according to the degree of displacement by **Garden's classification (I-IV).**
  - **Garden I and II** fractures are undisplaced and can be managed conservatively with bed rest. However, due to the risk of displacement ($\approx 30\%$) and subsequently AVN, these fractures are usually internally fixed using cannulated screws.
  - **Garden III and IV** fractures are displaced and associated with a high risk of AVN and non-union; they are therefore managed surgically with hemi-arthroplasty, i.e. Austin-Moore.

Risk factors for fractured neck of femur

- ○ **Factors affecting bone strength:** osteoporosis, oteomalacia, underlying bone disease (e.g. Paget's disease, tumours, sedentary lifestyle)
- ○ **Factors increasing the likelihood of falls:** increasing age, alcohol excess, impaired vision, confusion, dementia, epilepsy, arrhythmias, medication, i.e. hypnotics, steroids
- ○ **Other:** maternal family history, smoking

PERI-OPERATIVE MANAGEMENT OF #NOF
- Adequate analgesia.
- Fluid resuscitation.
- Thromboprophylaxis (TEDS + subcutaneous heparin).
- Antibiotic prophylaxis (usually at induction).
- Care of pressure areas, early mobilisation and rehabilitation.
- Bisphosphonates if indicated.

Femoral shaft fractures
Usually occur due to a high-energy impact, often in the context of polytrauma. If there is a history of minor trauma only, suspect a pathological fracture. Fractures can affect the proximal, mid-shaft or distal femur and are associated with high risk of complications such as DVT, ARDS, fat embolus and MODS; this is reduced with early fracture fixation.

MANAGEMENT (*see General fracture management* section above) Requires an ATLS™ approach, with reduction and fixation of the fracture with a traction splint (e.g. Thomas splint) initially, to reduce bleeding and pain, followed by definitive management of the fracture, e.g. intramedullary nailing and rehabilitation.

16.4. Injuries to the knee
Patellar dislocation
Dislocation usually occurs laterally as a result of direct or indirect trauma, i.e. a valgus force on an externally rotated knee.

MANAGEMENT Reduce (by extending the knee, while applying pressure laterally over the patella), follow-up with physiotherapy. Consider surgery, if recurrent.

Extensor mechanism injuries (i.e. patella, patella and quadriceps tendon)

CLINICAL FEATURES   Palpable soft tissue defect within the extensor compartment and inability to straight leg raise.

- **Patella fractures:** mostly follow a direct force; may be repaired surgically, e.g. with tension band wiring.
- **Tendon injuries:** usually arise due to sudden contraction of quadriceps on a flexed loaded knee.

Meniscal injuries

Commonly sports-related due to rotational injuries, or degenerative (in older patients).

CLINICAL FEATURES   Joint line pain; joint effusion (developing over hours); quadriceps femoris muscle disuse atrophy; locking (limiting knee extension) and giving way of the knee; and a positive McMurray's test.

MANAGEMENT   Joint effusion aspiration (to exclude infection); x-ray, MRI +/– arthroscopy. Treat with partial meniscectomy; intra-articular corticosteroids injection; analgesia and rehabilitation.

Anterior cruciate ligament (ACL) injury

Mechanisms of injury: hyperextension/rotational or twisting injuries, usually during sport, i.e. skiing, football. Incidence is greater in women.

CLINICAL FEATURES   Pain, joint instability and rapid swelling of the joint following injury (as ACL is highly vascular).

MANAGEMENT
Physiotherapy +/– open/arthroscopic reconstruction, in select cases.

Posterior cruciate ligament (PCL) injury

Mechanisms of injury: commonly, 'dashboard' injuries, where the proximal tibia is forced posteriorly relative to the distal femur.

CLINICAL FEATURES   Joint instability; rarely knee pain or swelling.

MANAGEMENT   Controversial – may involve ORIF or reconstruction, physiotherapy +/– use of supporting knee brace.

Collateral (medial + lateral) ligament injuries

Medial (MCL) and lateral (LCL) collateral ligament injuries are common and occur due to valgus and varus stresses on the knee, respectively; usually sports related.

CLINICAL FEATURES
- Knee swelling + erythema developing over several days.
- Pain and stiffness localised to the medial (MCL) or lateral (LCL) compartment.
- Positive valgus (MCL) or varus stress test (LCL).

MANAGEMENT   MRI to establish the extent of injury. Definitive treatment ranges from analgesia and early mobilisation to hinged knee bracing and early surgical repair.

Tibial fractures

The most common diaphyseal fracture in adults; can also affect the tibial plateau. Aetiology: mainly, motor vehicle accidents ($\approx$ 50% of cases) and sports related, i.e. football. Importantly, $\approx$ 25% are open and associated with extensive soft tissue loss.

MANAGEMENT   *See Fractures* section. Closed fractures can be treated conservatively with casts or functional bracing; open fractures require surgical fixation, i.e. with intramedullary nails, plates or frames. Common complications include non-union and compartment syndrome.

16.5. Important lower limb congenital disorders

Clubfoot (congenital talipes equinovarus)

Most common foot and ankle deformity in the UK. 3:1 male to female ratio; bilateral in 50% of cases.

CLINICAL FEATURES   Equinus and varus deviation of the foot with adduction of the forefoot. Importantly, assess for co-existing abnormalities of the hips and spine. Diagnosis is in-utero with ultrasound.

Aetiology of clubfoot

Primary (idiopathic): e.g. genetic, developmental arrest/delay
Secondary: e.g. spina bifida, neuromuscular disease (e.g. cerebral palsy)

MANAGEMENT
- Counselling.
- Treat within first week of life with manipulation and serial plaster casts or, continuous physiotherapy (i.e. stretching/counter-pressure).
- If conservative treatment fails, surgical correction is required.

Developmental dysplasia of the hip (DDH)

Described as instability or dysplasia of the hip joint. Otherwise known as Congenital Dislocation of the Hip (CDH). Three times more common in the left hip; bilateral in 10% of cases. Incidence is four times greater in girls and higher in Caucasians.

Aetiology of DDH

Unclear, thought to be due to familial and intra-uterine factors.
○ Familial (polygenic).
○ Hormonal: maternal hormones cross the placenta at birth leading to foetal hip laxity.
○ Birth factors: breech presentation, Caesarean section, first born, oligohydramnios, prematurity.

CLINICAL FEATURES
- Associated with other abnormalities, i.e. torticollis, scoliosis.
- Presentation can be within neonatal period or delayed, with:
  - wide perineum, asymmetric thigh creases, shortening of one thigh; Trendelenburg gait
  - Ortolani's manoeuvre (adduction to abduction of the flexed hip) + Barlow's test demonstrate reducible/irreducible dislocation and subluxation, respectively; form part of National screening programme at birth.

MANAGEMENT
- Imaging: ultrasound for diagnosis (more useful than x-ray as femoral head

+ acetabulum are composed of unossified cartilage) and also useful for monitoring disease +/– arthrography.
- Majority ($\approx 90\%$) stabilise by two weeks after birth without intervention.
- Treatment options include: abduction splint (e.g. Pavlik harness, hip spica) – used up to age 6–8 months; traction; open surgical reduction or closed manipulation.
- Family counselling – 10 fold risk of second child being affected.

16.6. Child with a limp

Most common cause of a painful limp in a child is trauma but other causes need to be excluded.

Differential diagnosis of an irritable hip

- ○ Trauma
- ○ Osteomyelitis of femur
- ○ Perthes' Disease
- ○ Tumours of bone/soft tissue
- ○ Septic arthritis
- ○ Transient synovitis
- ○ Slipped upper femoral epiphysis (SUFE)
- ○ Inflammatory arthritis
- ○ Secondary to abdominal pathology, i.e. psoas abscess, appendicitis

Transient synovitis

Most common non-traumatic cause of an irritable hip. Defined as a transient, non-specific synovitis of the hip, with effusion. Peak age: 3–8 years; male to female ratio is 2:1; can affect both hips.

CLINICAL FEATURES   Pain in the hip or thigh (referred pain), with stiffness often there is a history of preceding recent ear, upper respiratory or gastrointestinal tract infection. Child is reluctant to weight-bear with the hip held in flexion, abducted and externally rotated. Diagnosis is one of exclusion.

MANAGEMENT   Bed rest, analgesia (NSAIDs); occasionally traction. Condition is self-limiting.

Perthes' disease

Aseptic necrosis of all or part of the femoral head due to impairment of the blood supply by recurrent infarction; aetiology unknown. Can progress to avascular necrosis. Associated with long-term risk of developing early OA (in 30s) of the hip joint. Peak age: 3–9 years; 3–5 times more common in males; both hips affected in <10%.

CLINICAL FEATURES
- Examination can be normal.
- Positive findings include:
  - abnormal gait, positive Trendelenberg test
  - leg length discrepancy
  - restricted hip movement; as well as fixed flexion, external rotation and adduction deformities.

MANAGEMENT
- Investigations: x-ray ('frog-lateral' view).
- Treatment
  - conservative: analgesia; bimonthly follow-up; advise avoidance of contact sports and physiotherapy
  - surgical: $\approx 40\%$ will require surgery, i.e. osteotomy.

Slipped upper femoral epiphysis (SUFE)

'Slippage' of the epiphysis posteriorly and inferiorly. Can be bilateral. Peak incidence: 14–16 years in boys, 11–13 years in girls (i.e. pre-menarche). 3:1 male to female ratio.

CLINICAL FEATURES
- Antalgic limp + hip or knee pain, typically, in a pre-adolescent, obese male.
- On examination: inability to weight bear; antalgic or 'waddling' gait; limb shortening; restricted range of hip movements.

MANAGEMENT
- Investigations: x-ray (AP + lateral views) confirms diagnosis.
- Treatment includes reduction of the 'slip' with surgical fixation, i.e. in situ screw or osteotomy and rehabilitation. Consider prophylactic pinning of contralateral hip.

16.7. Osteomyelitis

This is an inflammatory reaction of bone in response to a pyogenic organism which, left untreated, will lead to irreversible destruction of the joint/limb. Can be classified according to: route of entry of the infecting pathogen (**exogenous**, i.e. following surgery or an open fracture, or **haematogenous** following bacteraemia); or time-course of the clinical presentation, i.e. **acute**, **subacute** or **chronic**. Complications of osteomyelitis: avascular necrosis, pathological fractures, chronic infection, growth disturbance (arrest, with shortening or angular deformity of the limb), septic arthritis.

AGE	PATHOGEN
Neonate	*Staph. aureus*; Group B *Streptococcus*; *E. Coli*
Infants or pre-school	*Staph. Aureus*; *Haemophilus influenzae*
>5 years – adult	*Staph. aureus*; *Salmonella* (assoc. with sickle cell), *Pseudomonas*, Fungi (chronically ill on long-term antibiotics)

CLINICAL FEATURES
- Risk factors: diabetes, immunocompromise (e.g. HIV, IgA deficiency), chronic illness, malnutrition, exposure to haematogenous source (dental procedure, abrasion, urethral catheterisation).
- Systemic symptoms: malaise and pyrexia.
- Local symptoms: point bony tenderness, limp (reluctance to weight-bear) or pseudoparalysis, muscle spasm +/– limited range of movements.

INVESTIGATIONS
- Blood tests: CRP, ESR and WCC elevated.
- X-ray: osseous changes are not evident in the first 7–10 days; in chronic osteomyelitis characteristic periosteal elevation and a sequestrum of dead bone surrounded by a sleeve of involucrum (new bone) may be seen +/– Brodie's abscess (seen as a cavity with sclerotic margins).
- MRI: 100% sensitive; detects early changes.
- Ultrasound: may show early subperiosteal oedema; useful for excluding an effusion.
- Bone scan: useful for differentiating multi- from unifocal infections.

MANAGEMENT
- Fluid resuscitation.
- Blood cultures followed by commencement of antibiotics, i.e. flucloxacillin + fucidin in adults and third generation cephalosporins in children <5 years old.
- Aspiration of joint if appropriate – send aspirate for urgent Gram stain and MC&S.
- Analgesia +/– splinting of the affected limb.
- Surgical options: soft tissue/abscess drainage +/– biopsy (for histology and microbiology) +/– sequestrectomy and bone grafting in chronic osteomyelitis.

16.8. Bone tumours
Can be primary or secondary, i.e. metastatic.

Metastatic bone tumours
Commonly arise from prostate, breast, kidney, lung and thyroid primaries. Rarely, skin (e.g. melanoma). Spread is haematogenous. The spine, long bones, pelvis and ribs are the most frequently affected sites. Lesions are typically *lytic* with the exception of prostatic metastases, which are *sclerotic*.

CLINICAL FEATURES
- Can be asymptomatic (in early stages) and may be discovered following diagnosis of the primary tumour.
- ≈ 50% develop symptoms: constant bone pain; antalgic/altered gait; pathological fractures (commonly of the femur, humerus and spine).
- Spinal deposits +/– spinal instability or cord compression.
- Hypercalcaemia.

MANAGEMENT
- Involves treatment of:
  - primary malignancy
  - symptoms: e.g. analgesia for bony pain +/– radiotherapy
  - complications: e.g. hypercalcaemia and fractures (with bisphosphonates +/– prophylactic fixation of bones at risk).

Malignant primary bone tumours
Rare. Accounts for 0.5% of all tumours. Often misdiagnosed. Evaluation requires careful history, examination (including the breasts in women and prostate in men), investigation and staging.

CLINICAL FEATURES
Include bony pain (typically worse with activity and at night), restricted movement of adjacent joints and pathological fractures. Can be asymptomatic. Examination may reveal a limp (if lower limb affected) and the presence of a painless soft tissue mass.

INVESTIGATIONS
- Imaging may include:
  - plain x-ray of affected bone
  - MRI/CT of the bone involved
  - whole body MRI, technetium bone scanning
  - ultrasound and mammography (in females)
  - chest x-ray (for metastases; only useful if mass >2 cm) or chest CT scan.

- Blood tests: FBC, CRP, ESR, calcium, phosphate, ALP, serum PSA in males, serum and urine protein electrophoresis (for myeloma).

MANAGEMENT
- Medical: primarily chemotherapy.
- Surgical options include curretage/wide excision of primary tumour +/− limb reconstruction; excision of pulmonary metastases; amputation.

Differential diagnosis for bone tumours

AGE 0–5 YEARS	AGE 5–20 YEARS	AGE 20–40 YEARS	>40 YEARS
Osteomyelitis	Bone cyst	Ewing's sarcoma	Metastases
Metastastatic neuroblastoma	Osteosarcoma	Giant cell tumour	Myeloma/lymphoma
Leukaemia	Ewing's sarcoma	Osteosarcoma Spindle cell tumours	Chondrosarcoma
	Osteomyelitis	Chondrosarcoma	Osteosarcoma due to Paget's/irradiation

Osteosarcoma
- Rapidly-growing tumour; metastasises early; 5-year survival 60–65%. Majority occur between the ages of 10–25 years; 1.5:1 male to female ratio.
- Characteristically found in metaphysis of long bones (especially around knee).
- ALP typically elevated (prognostic indicator).
- Management: wide excision +/− limb reconstruction + chemotherapy.

Chondrosarcoma
- Second most common primary bone tumour; onset between 30–70 years.
- Can arise in long or flat bones, i.e. pelvis, scapula.
- Treatment: wide local resection; local recurrence common.

Ewing's sarcoma
- Small round cell tumour of bone; majority occur <20 years old; more common in males; 5-year survival about 50%.
- Typically, affects diaphysis of long and flat bones.
- Characteristic 'onion-skin' (periosteal elevation) appearance + soft tissue mass on imaging.
- Management: chemotherapy, tumour resection +/− post-operative radiotherapy.

Spindle cell sarcomas
- Includes: fibrosarcomas, malignant fibrous histiocytomas and leiomyosarcomas.
- Treatment and prognosis similar to osteosarcomas.

16.9. Short cases in orthopaedics
Dupuytren's disease
Benign condition, where nodular fibromatosis of the palmar or plantar fascia leads to permanent and often progressive contracture of the associated digit. Aetiology is unknown but can be familial or associated with previous hand trauma, phenytoin, alcohol, diabetes mellitus.

CLINICAL FEATURES   Presents with deformity and loss of hand/foot function; the ring finger, little finger and middle finger are most commonly affected. Bilateral in 65% of cases.

MANAGEMENT   Consider steroid injections, splints and surgical excision of the affected fascia. Recurrence rates are high.

Ganglion
A benign cystic swelling arising from a joint or tendon sheath; contents resemble synovial fluid. 3:1 male to female ratio. Causes: trauma, joint overuse, or idiopathic.

MANAGEMENT   If symptomatic, aspiration (≈ 50% recur) or surgical excision followed by immobilisation of the joint for 1–2 weeks.

Trigger finger/thumb (aka tenosynovitis)
Painful locking of the thumb or finger which is functionally limiting. Thought to be due to focal degeneration within the flexor tendon sheath, leading to localised inflammation and limiting movement of the tendon within its sheath. 1:4 male to female ratio.

CLINICAL FEATURES   Palpable nodule in the distal palm which moves with flexion and extension; triggering or locking at the MCP/DIP joint which in later stages requires release by passive manipulation using the other hand +/– clicking or crepitus.

MANAGEMENT   Splinting, corticosteroid injection or surgical release.

Tennis elbow (aka lateral epicondylitis)
The most common cause of elbow pain.

CLINICAL FEATURES   Pain and tenderness over the lateral epicondyle radiating down forearm, typically exacerbated by wrist extension.

MANAGEMENT   NSAIDs and physiotherapy, or surgical release of the extensor origin at the elbow, if conservative treatment fails.

Golfer's elbow (aka medial epicondylitis)
Pain over the medial epicondyle exacerbated by resisted pronation of the forearm and wrist flexion.

MANAGEMENT   NSAIDs and physiotherapy, or surgical release of the flexor origin at the elbow in a few cases.

Charcot's joint (aka neuropathic joint)
Chronic, progressive, destructive arthropathy. Causes: chronic neuropathies, e.g. diabetes, syringomyelia (and traditionally infection such as syphilis and leprosy).

CLINICAL FEATURES   Loss of pain and proprioceptive sensation. The foot, ankle and knee are commonly affected.

MANAGEMENT   Treat the underlying cause; advise and educate regarding protection of the joint; surgery – rarely, usually reserved for severe disease.

Ophthalmology

17.1. Painful red eye

Beware that eyesight may be threatened and action may be required immediately. Causes:

- **Conjunctivitis (bacterial, viral or allergic):** mild discomfort and irritation (severe pain should alert you to other possible causes) with discharge (purulent suggests a bacterial cause, whereas viral is associated with a watery discharge). Eyes are itchy in allergic conjunctivitis.
- **Keratitis (bacterial, viral, fungal or protozoal):** i.e. inflammation of the cornea. May cause severe pain, reduced vision and discharge (which may be watery, mucoid or purulent). There may be ulceration: this threatens eyesight and is an emergency – refer to ophthalmologists immediately. Causes: *Staphylococcus* or *Pseudomonas* (bacterial), HSV (viral – causes 'dendritic' ulcers), acanthamoeba (protozoal – more common in contact lens wearers).
- **Episcleritis: produces** normally only mild discomfort and self-limiting.
- **Scleritis:** more severe pain than episcleritis and commonly associated with systemic disease, e.g. rheumatoid arthritis. Patient may also complain of reduced vision.
- **Anterior uveitis:** *see* below.
- **Trauma to the cornea/foreign body**.
- **Acute glaucoma** – *see* below.

Note: some of the causes above more commonly cause minor irritation or mild discomfort, e.g. conjunctivitis, episcleritis. Other causes of a red eye (usually painless) include subconjunctival haemorrhage and blepharitis.

17.2. Unilateral sudden loss of vision

It is important to distinguish between painless versus painful (identified in brackets) causes.

- Acute glaucoma (painful).
- Vitreous haemorrhage.
- Central retinal artery occlusion (pale retina with 'cherry red' spot).
- Central retinal vein occlusion.
- Retinal detachment.

- Age-related macular degeneration (usually gradual but can be sudden).
- Anterior ischaemic optic neuropathy.
- Temporal arteritis.
- Non-arteritic.
- Optic neuritis (painful).

17.3. Uveitis
Inflammation of the uveal tract, i.e. the iris, ciliary body and choroid.

Anterior uveitis (iritis)
Associated with systemic disease in ≈ 50% cases, e.g. sarcoidosis, seronegative arthritis, Behcet's disease.

CLINICAL FEATURES   Can present acutely as a painful red eye with blurred vision and photophobia or more chronically with milder symptoms. A hypopyon may be present and there may be keratic precipitates (clumps of inflammatory cells) and synechiae (adhesions of the iris to the lens).

TREATMENT   With topical steroids, and drops to dilate the pupil (e.g. cyclopentolate) to prevent synechiae (adhesions of iris to lens).

Posterior uveitis
- Normally presents with blurred vision without pain or red eye.
- May be associated with systemic disease, e.g. toxoplasmosis or Behcet's disease.

17.4. Cataracts
Opacity of the lens. Incidence increases with age.

CLINICAL FEATURES   Gradual painless loss of vision with glare; with loss of the red reflex on fundoscopy. Associated with:
- Increasing age.
- Ocular disease, e.g. high myopia.
- Systemic disease, e.g. diabetes, myotonic dystrophy.
- Drugs, e.g. steroids.

MANAGEMENT   Surgery if symptoms affect quality of life.

17.5. Glaucoma
Damage to the optic nerve secondary to raised intraocular pressure. Classified as primary or secondary (associated with ocular disease); acute or chronic; and closed-angle (iris in contact with the trabecular meshwork) or open-angle (iris not in contact with the trabecular meshwork):
- Chronic (open angle) – asymptomatic until well-advanced but causes progressive visual field defect with cupped optic disc; routine screening necessary for early diagnosis; familial – check relatives. Treatment: with topical eye drops, e.g. latanoprost, β-blockers (e.g. timolol), pilocarpine. Rarely surgery is necessary – trabeculectomy.
- Acute closed angle – presents with painful, red eye with loss of vision. Pupil may be fixed and dilated. Urgent treatment is required with IV acetazolamide, topical pilocarpine and then laser iridotomy or iridectomy.

17.6. Retinal disease
Diabetic retinopathy
Occurs in virtually all type I diabetics after 15–20 years and 80% of type II diabetics ($\approx$ 10% at diagnosis and 50% at 10 years). Commonest cause of blindness in developed world in 30–60 year olds. Normally classified as:

- Background: microaneurysms; dot, blot and flame haemorrhages; hard exudates.
- Pre-proliferative: as for background + cotton wool spots; dilation and beading of veins; and intraretinal microvascular abnormalities (IRMAs).
- Proliferative: neovascularisation, vitreous haemorrhage, retinal detachment, glaucoma (rubeosis iridis).

Maculopathy = retinopathy involving the macula, therefore likely to cause visual loss even with less severe disease: typically causes poor central vision with relatively intact peripheral vision.

Patients need good glycaemic control but other management depends on the type:

- Background: monitor for progression.
- Pre-proliferative: monitor closely +/– panretinal laser photocoagulation in some circumstances.
- Proliferative: panretinal laser photocoagulation.
- Maculopathy: focal laser photocoagulation.

Note: that patients with diabetes are also more likely to develop glaucoma and cataracts.

Hypertensive retinopathy
Associated with compensated hypertension (often called grades 1 and 2):

- 1: 'copper' or 'silver' wiring (attenuation of the arterioles).
- 2: AV nipping.

Associated with accelerated hypertension (often called grades 3 and 4):

- 3: flame haemorrhages, cotton wool spots, hard exudates.
- 4: papilloedema.

Age-related macular degeneration
Commonest cause of blindness in over 65s in the developed world: normally gradual loss of central vision with peripheral vision intact. Two types: dry or non-exudative (presence of lipid deposits or drusen) and the more severe wet or exudative (new vessel formation causing a subretinal neovascular membrane).

Retinitis pigmentosa
Hereditary condition with clinical features of night blindness, tunnel vision and classical fundus appearance (bone-spicule pigmentation, pale disc, attenuated blood vessels).

18

Ear, nose and throat

18.1. Disorders of the ear
18.2. Disorders of the nose and throat

18.1. Disorders of the ear
Hearing loss
- Conductive, i.e. due to pathology in the middle or outer ear.
- Sensorineural, i.e. due to pathology in the cochlea or auditory nerve.
- Mixed conductive/sensorineural.

Causes of conductive hearing loss
○ Wax (although wax impaction has to be very severe to cause hearing loss)
○ Otitis media (acute, chronic or with effusion)
○ Perforation
○ Cholesteatoma
○ Otosclerosis

Causes of sensorineural hearing loss
○ Presbycusis
○ Noise-induced
○ Ménière's disease (although vertigo is more of a problem in this condition)
○ Congenital, e.g. maternal rubella infection
○ Drugs, e.g. aminoglyosides
○ Infections, e.g. mumps
○ Acoustic neuroma

Otitis externa
Infection of the external meatus, most commonly bacterial, e.g. *Staph.* or *Pseudomonas*. Clinical features: pain and tenderness over the ear, mild discharge, and sometimes deafness. Treatment: short course of topical antibiotics generally effective.

Otitis media (OM)
Inflammation of the middle ear.

Acute
Normally follows an URTI (either viral or bacterial), frequently bilateral and most common in children. Clinical features: ear pain/tenderness, conductive deafness, fever and an abnormal ear drum on otoscopy (e.g. bulging, redness, perforation with otorrhoea). Management: many will resolve spontaneously but if not, antibiotic therapy should be started.

Chronic suppurative (CSOM)

Failure of acute OM to resolve may lead to chronic OM with persistent discharge and worsening deafness. Classified as active (presence of infection) or inactive, and by whether there is a perforation or presence of cholesteatoma (growth of squamous epithelium in the middle ear). Complications are classified as intratemporal (e.g. ossicular erosion, facial nerve palsy) or intracranial (e.g. meningitis, brain abscess).

With effusion ('glue ear')

Collection of serous or viscous fluid in the middle ear. Very common in children, causing conductive deafness and mild ear discomfort. Ear drum is usually abnormal on examination (e.g. dull or immobile).

MANAGEMENT If it does not spontaneously resolve, consider adenoidectomy +/– myringotomy and grommet insertion. Occurs rarely in adults when it may be a sign of a nasopharyngeal cancer – therefore important to examine post-nasal space with nasendoscope (or mirror).

18.2. Disorders of the nose and throat

Sinusitis

Inflammation of the mucous membranes of the paranasal sinuses. More commonly acute but in a small proportion of cases which do not resolve, it becomes chronic. Usually related to an URTI (viral or bacterial) but in some cases will follow dental infection.

CLINICAL FEATURES Include nasal obstruction, post-nasal drip, headache or pain over the sinuses.

MANAGEMENT Acute treatment with intranasal decongestants to facilitate sinus drainage and if it does not resolve spontaneously then appropriate antibiotics should be given; in chronic disease, washout or surgery may be necessary.

Epistaxis

Very common but usually self-limiting and does not require medical intervention. The site of bleeding is commonly Little's area (a plexus of vessels on the anterior part of the nasal septum). Normally no cause is identified but causes include trauma, clotting disorders and anticoagulant therapy.

Severe epistaxis is an emergency!

- ○ ABC important, particularly management of the airway. Patients may need IV fluids +/– blood if very severe (also check FBC, clotting and cross-match)
- ○ Sit patient up with head leant forward; if simple compression or nasal plugging does not help and bleeding is persistent – options include cautery (with silver nitrate), nasal packing (e.g. anteriorly with nasal tampons or bismuth, iodoform and paraffin paste (BIPP) or if posterior can use Foley catheter), or rarely surgery (e.g. arterial ligation +/– neuroradiological embolisation)
- ○ Patient may need admission if elderly and persistent bleeding

Tonsillitis – inflammation of the tonsils

Acute tonsillitis

CLINICAL FEATURES   Include sore throat, referred ear pain, headache, fever and malaise. Tonsils are enlarged and may exude pus. There may be cervical lymphadenopathy. Causes: viruses or bacteria (particularly *Streptococcus pyogenes*).

MANAGEMENT   Most patients will improve without antibiotics. If recurrent (>7 per year or >5 in two years) then tonsillectomy is indicated.

Quinsy (peritonsillar abscess)

A complication of acute (usually Streptococcal) tonsillitis. Should be suspected if a patient with acute tonsillitis deteriorates with referred ear pain, dysphagia and trismus.

MANAGEMENT   Systemic penicillin and surgical drainage is necessary acutely, and consideration of tonsillectomy.

Epiglottitis

Occurs most commonly in children. Causes: *Haem. influenzae* (and therefore less common now because of HIb vaccine).

CLINICAL FEATURES   Child presents with general malaise, dysphagia, 'quack-like' cough and then stridor. **Acute epiglottitis is an emergency** as there is a danger of airway obstruction – very urgent ENT review (and an experienced anesthetist) will be needed – important not to look in throat as this can precipitate obstruction.

Breast disease

19.1. Mastalgia

Breast pain is common and can be cyclical (mean age 33 years) or non-cyclical (mean age 45 years). Causes include periductal mastitis, fat necrosis, sclerosing adenosis, Tietze's syndrome (costochondritis) and rarely, breast cancer.

Management requires exclusion of underlying breast cancer; lifestyle modification (e.g. low saturated fat diets, weight loss, caffeine reduction); supportive bra; medical treatment (e.g. evening primrose oil, danazol (GnRH inhibitor) or bromocriptine (inhibits prolactin release) in severe cases); and analgesia, e.g. NSAIDs.

19.2. Nipple discharge

May arise from a single or multiple ducts and can be categorised by aetiology:
- Physiological: intermittent, spontaneous yellow/brown/green/white discharge. Common in multiparous females. Treat conservatively.
- Duct ectasia (*see* below).
- Periductal mastitis: affects younger women and is associated with smoking. Can be unilateral or bilateral with symptoms similar to duct ectasia, however, the nipple discharge is typically offensive. *Staph. aureus*, Enterococci, anaerobic Streptococci and *Bacteroides* are most commonly implicated. Treat with appropriate antibiotics and advise smoking cessation.
- Intraductal papilloma – *see* below.
- Galactorrhoea: bilateral discharge of milk not associated with breast-feeding. Causes are those that lead to hyperprolactinaemia, e.g. dopamine antagonists, pituitary adenoma, Cushing's disease and hypothyroidism. Management involves treatment of the underlying cause +/– dopamine receptor agonist, e.g. bromocriptine.

19.3. Breast lumps: overview

May be benign or malignant. All patients presenting with a breast lump should undergo triple assessment:
- History and examination.
- Radiological: ultrasound if <35 years; mammogram if >35 years; MRI in select cases.

- Pathological: fine needle aspiration for cytology (FNAC) +/− core biopsy for grading (*see* below) and oestrogen receptor positivity.

FNAC classification

- ○ C1: Inadequate
- ○ C2: Normal
- ○ C3: Atypia probably benign
- ○ C4: Atypia probably malignant
- ○ C5: Malignant

19.4. Benign breast lumps

Benign mammary dysplasia (fibrocystic change, fibroadenosis or benign breast disease)

Common. Occurs between ages 35–45 years. Thought to be due to a hormonal imbalance, e.g. peri-menopause.

CLINICAL FEATURES   Characterised by a fluctuating (cyclical), painful lump, nodularity or cysts.

MANAGEMENT   Reassurance, aspiration (if cyst), supportive bra, analgesia +/− evening primrose oil or rarely, danazol/bromocriptine.

Fibroadenoma

Common. Typically occurs in young women. Hormone related – often presents in the second half of menstrual cycle.

CLINICAL FEATURES   Painless, mobile hard lump, small and well circumscribed with a lobulated surface (so-called 'breast mice').

MANAGEMENT   If age <22 years, observe, may regress; if age >22 years, consider excision.

Breast abscess

Can be lactational or non-lactational (*see* periductal mastitis above). *Staph. aureus*, *Staph. epidermidis* and Streptococci are most commonly implicated in the latter, with the majority occurring within six weeks of childbirth.

MANAGEMENT   Treat early with antibiotics +/− aspiration or incision and drainage.

Ductal ectasia (plasma cell mastitis)

Sterile inflammation due to ductal involution. Typically presents in peri-menopausal women with pain (cyclical), erythema +/− subareolar lump and black/green/grey nipple discharge and nipple inversion. Usually bilateral.

MANAGEMENT   Treat conservatively with analgesia and supportive bra – usually settles within 3–4 weeks; consider curative duct excision in severe cases.

Fat necrosis

Rare. Typically follows surgery or trauma.

CLINICAL FEATURES   Presents as a hard, irregular lump +/– tethering. Calcification may be seen on mammography.

MANAGEMENT   Analgesia +/– excision for pain control.

Haematoma
Typically follows trauma, however, may be spontaneous. *Note*: it can be the initial presentation of underlying breast carcinoma.

Intraductal papilloma
A benign neoplasm of the ductal epithelium. Associated with a 1–2 fold risk of developing breast cancer. Typically presents with bloody nipple discharge.

MANAGEMENT   Requires surgical excision of the affected duct, i.e. microdochectomy, once carcinoma has been excluded.

Phylloides tumour
Rare. Typically fast-growing fibroepithelial tumour; affects those >35 years old. Usually benign but can undergo malignant sarcomatous transformation. Treatment is with wide local excision or mastectomy.

19.5. Breast cancer
Most common cancer in young women. Diagnosis is made following triple assessment. Risk factors include early menarche, late menopause (>54 years), nulliparity, family history (BRCA1/2 carriers have a 50% risk by age 50 years), drugs (HRT, OCP), irradiation, commoner in social class I and II. Screening: women over 50 years are invited for mammography 3-yearly until the age of 70 years.

CLINICAL FEATURES
- Lump: typically painless, irregular and craggy.
- Nipple discharge (often bloody).
- Nipple inversion (due to underlying lesion) and skin changes: tethering, dimpling, erythema/eczema (Paget's disease), peau d'orange and ulceration (a late sign).

INVESTIGATIONS
- Triple assessment (*see* above).
- Investigation for metastatic disease if clinically indicated, e.g. CXR, ultrasound/CT of the pelvis/abdomen, bone scan, PET scan.

Histological types – *can be in situ or invasive*
- ○ **Ductal carcinoma in situ:** Pre-malignant condition. Typically affects peri- or post-menopausal women and usually impalpable, i.e. detected at screening. Associated with 30–50% risk of developing invasive cancer at 10 years. Microcalcification is commonly seen at mammography and diagnosis is made following stereo-guided biopsy. Ductal carcinoma involving the nipple is known as Paget's disease of the nipple
- ○ **Invasive ductal carcinoma:** Ductal carcinoma is graded 1 to 3 (1= low-grade, 3= high-grade and poorly differentiated); classically, a stellate mass with microcalcification is seen on mammography
- ○ **Lobular carcinoma in situ:** Commonly affects pre-menopausal women and 70% are multi-focal and/or bilateral. Associated with a 15–20% risk of developing invasive breast cancer at 10 years

MANAGEMENT   Options for management depend on histological grade and stage and include:

- Wide local excision (WLE) or mastectomy +/– axillary lymph node clearance for local control +/– adjuvant radiotherapy +/– chemotherapy.
- In addition, hormone therapy, e.g. oestrogen receptor antagonists, such as tamoxifen and aromatase inhibitors, such as anastrazole, may also prove beneficial in oestrogen receptor positive cancers in post-menopausal women.
- If late presentation, treatment is palliative, e.g. analgesia, radiotherapy (for bony pain relief).

20

Peri-operative care

20.1. Pre-operative assessment

Pre-operative assessment establishes whether a patient can tolerate the physiological stresses of anaesthesia and surgery and more accurately assesses individual risk in the context of pre-existing or intercurrent disease. Moreover, it facilitates pre-optimisation of the patient and enables peri-operative care to be tailored to the individual with the anticipation of post-operative requirements such as HDU/ITU. Assessment usually occurs in an outpatient setting and involves a comprehensive history, examination and appropriate investigations with referral to a specialist, e.g. cardiologist, as required.

Factors associated with increased peri-operative risk

- Age >60 years
- CCF
- Previous CABG
- Diabetes mellitus
- COPD
- Neurological disease
- BMI <20 or >35
- IHD
- Peripheral vascular disease
- Renal failure
- Pulmonary and arterial hypertension

Medical co-morbidity increases the risk associated with anaesthesia and surgery. In addition to establishing current health, an anaesthetic history should be performed. This includes:

- Previous anaesthetic complications.
- Family history of anaesthetic complications, (e.g. due to porphyria, pseudocholinesterase deficiency, malignant hyperpyrexia).
- Airway/neck problems (RA, ankylosing spondylosis, trauma with C-spine immobilization).
- Drug history (anticoagulation/antiplatelets); allergies (latex/antibiotics).
- Cultural beliefs (i.e. Jehovah's Witness) that may impact on peri-operative care should also be established and documented.

PRE-OPERATIVE INVESTIGATIONS These can be categorised into those that aid diagnosis or planning (CT scanning, barium enema), and those that are 'routine.' The latter include blood tests (FBC, U&E, LFTs, clotting, glucose, tests for sickle cell disease), CXR, ECG, urinalysis, arterial blood gas, lung function tests, echocardiography as well as more specialist investigations.

The operative procedure, classified into minor/intermediate, major, major+ or complex and the patient's ASA grading in conjunction with the patient's pre-operative comorbidity/physical status, will influence the investigations requested.

American Society of Anaesthetists grading system (ASA)

Grade

I   A normal healthy patient (no significant co-morbidity or medical history)
II   A patient with mild systemic disease, with no functional limitation
III   A patient with moderate systemic disease with functional limitations
IV   A patient with severe systemic disease that is a constant threat to life
V   Moribund patient who is not expected to survive another 24 hours with or without surgery
VI   Brain-dead patient whose organs being removed for donation
E   Emergency

50% of patients for elective surgery are ASA grade 1.

ASA 1 is associated with an operative mortality of < 1: 10 000; this rises to approx. 50% for ASA V.

20.2. Peri-operative fluid management

Total body water equates to approximately 60% of total body weight in a man ($\approx$ 55% in a woman). A 70 kg male is therefore composed of approximately 42 litres of water of which:

- (28 litres) is **Intracellular.**
- (14 litres) is **Extracellular** – this can be divided into 2 further compartments:
  - **intravascular:** i.e. plasma 1/4 (3.5 litres)
  - **extravascular** compartment: 3/4 – composed of **interstitial** (10.5 litres) and **transcellular** fluid spaces (0.5 litres) e.g. CSF, peritoneal, ocular and synovial fluid.

Fluid Balance

Refers to the net fluid intake and output from the body; an excessive loss results in a negative balance; an excessive intake results in a positive balance.

In a healthy 70 kg male:
- ○ **Overall Fluid Intake** (2500 ml) = oral fluid ($\approx$ 1200 ml) + metabolic (water produced by body $\approx$ 300 ml) + food (1000 ml)
- ○ **Overall Fluid Output** (2500 ml) = urine ($\approx$1500 ml) + stool ($\approx$ 300 ml) + insensible losses (lung and skin 600-900 ml)

Fluid Therapy

The purpose of fluid therapy is to correct both normal and abnormal fluid as well as electrolyte losses, thereby restoring intravascular fluid volume, BP and thus tissue oxygenation. An accurate assessment (i.e. history and examination) of fluid balance is therefore essential. It is a good idea to calculate the:

1   DEFICIT, i.e. starvation time
2   LOSS, i.e. intra-operative blood loss
3   Maintenance fluids required ($\approx$ 40 ml/kg/24 hrs).

CLINICAL FEATURES
- Tachycardia, hypotension, reduced skin turgor, dry mucous membranes, sunken eyes suggest dehydration.
- Evidence of third space loss (e.g. ascites, ankle oedema) suggests fluid is collecting within the wrong compartment.
- Urine output (UO) is a valuable indicator of end-organ perfusion: oliguria (UO <0.5 ml/kg/hr), anuria, concentrated urine suggests a need for fluid resuscitation.

Indications for fluid supplementation
- Insufficient oral intake: e.g. NBM
- Excessive fluid loss: e.g. diarrhoea, intra-operative blood loss, ileostomy/fistula output, vomiting, drain outputs, fever, burns, third space loss, e.g. ileus, ascites

Types of fluid
Crystalloids
- Isotonic solutions (e.g. 0.9% NaCl) are distributed evenly throughout the extracellular compartment
- Hypotonic solutions (e.g. 5% dextrose) are distributed throughout both the intra- and extracellular compartments

Colloids – useful in resuscitation scenario
- Exert a greater oncotic pressure and are retained to a greater extent within the intravascular compartment. Examples: human albumin, synthetic solutions including dextrans, gelatins (e.g. Haemaccel, Gelofusin), hydroxyethyl starches (e.g. Hespan)

Fluid regimens
In summary, daily basal requirement is 30–40 ml/kg of water, 1–2 mmol/kg of sodium and 1 mmol/kg of potassium.
On average, an adult will therefore require ≈ 3 litres of fluid, 60 mmol K^+ and 70–140 mmol Na^+ per day. There are a number of ways that this may be achieved:
- 3 L dextrose-saline with 20 mmol KCl in each bag; each running over 8 hours.
- 2 L 5% dextrose-saline + 1 L Normal saline with 20 mmol KCl in each bag; each over 8 hours.

20.3. Nutrition
More than 50% of patients in hospital are under-nourished. Factors implicated include:
- **Poor oral intake** (due to anorexia, nausea and vomiting, pain, inability to swallow; malabsorption (i.e. diarrhoea, pancreatic insufficiency, Crohn's disease, bowel resection).
- **Increased nutritional demand** (in response to surgery, burns, sepsis, cancer).
- **Increased nutrient loss** (high output fistulae/stoma/drains).

Poor nutrition becomes apparent when there is unintentional weight loss of >10% and is associated with increased post-operative mortality and morbidity, e.g. poor wound healing and infections. Nutritional assessment of all patients is therefore essential. Nutritional requirements depend on a number of factors: gender, weight, activity, pre-existing malnutrition, type of surgery and presence of infection. On average, a critically ill patient requires 25–30 kcal/kg/day.

Methods of assessing nutrition include weight (change), Body Mass Index (BMI), mid-arm circumference (assessment of muscle mass), triceps skinfold thickness (assessment of fat), food chart (assesses oral intake) and specific blood tests (serum albumin, pre-albumin and transferrin).

Indications for nutritional support
○ Prophylactically in the severely malnourished
○ If fasting/NBM/poor oral intake anticipated >7days
○ Increased nutritional demand not met by oral intake

Routes of administration
Enteral
This is the preferred route as it is easier to manage, with fewer complications and cheaper than parenteral nutrition. Feeds can be administered via a nasogastric tube (NGT), percutaneous endoscopic gastrostomy (PEG) or feeding jejenostomy tube. Indications include: in the unconscious patient, if unsafe swallow (e.g. following stroke) anorexia/poor oral intake, maxillofacial surgery/trauma, proximal GI obstruction/surgery. *Note*: if the patient is safe for oral intake then high-energy drinks can be provided (e.g. Calogen) to avoid more aggressive feeding options.

Complications of enteral nutrition
○ **NG tube:** malposition, displacement, blockage of the tube, oesophageal/gastric ulceration
○ **PEG tube:** pain, bleeding, peritonitis, infection and tube blockage or displacement
○ **Feed:** diarrhoea, aspiration, reflux, hyper-/hypoglycaemia, fluid overload or dehydration

Total Parenteral Nutrition (TPN)
Used if the enteral route is contraindicated, e.g. post-op ileus, colitis, short bowel syndrome, acute pancreatitis, intestinal obstruction, or perforation and is of little benefit if used for less than seven days. Due to the high osmolality of the feed and risk of thrombophlebitis, a central venous line is preferable.

Complications of TPN
○ **Related to line insertion:** e.g. pneumothorax, haemothorax, arterial puncture, failure of insertion
○ **Line related:** e.g. infection, blockage, venous thrombosis, thrombophlebitis (in peripheries)
○ **Feed related:** e.g. hyper-/hypoglycaemia, electrolyte abnormalities, refeeding syndrome, osteoporosis, hepatic dysfunction, e.g. cholestatic jaundice

20.4. Post-operative complications
Post-operative complications can be classified as **general** or **specific** to the type of operation performed or according to their time of onset:
● **Immediate** (occurring within the first 24 hours).
● **Early** (occurring within one month of surgery).
● **Late** (>1 month from surgery).

General complications
Immediate
● Pain.
● Nausea and vomiting +/– aspiration – related to the anaesthetic or analgesia.
● Primary haemorrhage, i.e. bleeding at the time of surgery.

- Basal atelectasis – may progress to a lower respiratory tract infection (LRTI).
- Shock (commonly hypovolaemic but may also be septic or cardiogenic).

Early
- Acute confusional state: e.g. due to hypoxia, pain, sepsis, metabolic abnormalities, dehydration, hypoglycaemia, alcohol withdrawal.
- Fever (low-grade <38° is common in the first 48 hours).
- Secondary haemorrhage: e.g. due to infection, ulceration or malignancy.
- Respiratory complications: pneumonia, ARDS, aspiration pneumonitis – may require antibiotics, physiotherapy, nebulisers, bronchoscopy +/– ventilation.
- DVT typically occurs at day six post-op; may be complicated by PE.
- Wound dehiscence or anastamotic leak (usually between day 7–10).
- Acute urinary retention.
- Urinary tract infection (UTI).
- Acute renal failure may be related to inadequate fluid resuscitation, contrast.
- Gastric stasis or paralytic ileus: more common following abdominal surgery; treatment includes NBM, NG tube + correction of electrolyte disturbances.
- Wound infection.

Late
- Incisional hernia.
- Bowel obstruction secondary to adhesions (following abdominal surgery).

MANAGEMENT Aimed at primary prevention and employs pre-emptive strategies such as DVT prophylaxis, adequate analgesia, aggressive fluid resuscitation both intra- and post-operatively, early mobilisation, nutritional support, etc. In addition to close monitoring in the post-operative phase, i.e. BP, heart rate, urine output, drain output, blood testing (FBC, U&Es, clotting).

Post-operative complications should be anticipated, detected early and managed appropriately.

20.5. Acute post-operative pain management
Pain is defined as an unpleasant sensory and emotional experience associated with actual or potential tissue damage, or described in terms of such damage.

Methods of assessing pain
- Verbal Rating Score, i.e. no pain, mild/moderate/severe pain
- Numerical Rating Score, i.e. 1 (no pain) to 10 (the worst pain imaginable)
- Visual Analogue Scale, i.e. where the patient indicates the intensity of their pain on a 10 cm graduated line
- Magill Pain Questionnaire – a multi-dimensional, complex form rarely used to assess acute pain

Post-operative pain is notoriously poorly managed and this has a number of important physiological and psychological consequences. Adverse effects of pain include reduced mobility (with increased risk of DVT) and, particularly in upper abdominal and thoracic surgery, reduced vital capacity and cough inhibition leading to retention of secretions, collapse of alveoli and an increased risk of atelectasis and LRTI.

World Health Organization (WHO) analgesic pain ladder
This provides a useful step-wise approach to managing pain irrespective of its origin.

Simple analgesics (e.g. paracetamol)
○ Used to treat mild to moderate pain and in combination with other analgesics in severe pain

Non-Steroidal Anti-inflammatory Drugs (NSAIDs, e.g. ibuprofen, diclofenac)
○ Used to treat mild to moderate pain and in combination with other drugs in severe pain; have an opioid sparing effect
○ Routes of administration: oral, intramuscularl or per rectal
○ *Note:* use with care in the elderly (risk of gastric ulceration)
○ Contra-indications include asthma, renal impairment and peptic ulceration

Weak opioids (e.g. codeine phosphate, dihydrocodeine, tramadol)

Strong opioids (e.g. morphine, pethidine, fentanyl)
○ Can be administered via a number of routes: subcutaneous, intramuscular, transdermal, intravenous and via a PCA (patient controlled analgesia). PCA analgesia has the advantage of improving patient autonomy, reducing nursing workload, and reducing fluctuations in plasma concentrations of drug
○ Side effects include sedation, nausea and vomiting, constipation, urinary retention, pruritis, respiratory depression

Local anaesthetics

Local anaesthetic (LA) agents (e.g. lidocaine) are useful for post-operative pain control and can be administered via several routes: local wound infiltration, nerve/plexus blocks. Importantly, LA has a maximum weight-dependent dose. Overdose can lead to convulsions and cardiac arrhythmias. *Note:* do not use LA with adrenaline for extremities, e.g. finger, nose, as adrenaline causes vasoconstriction and may lead to ischaemia of the extremity involved.

20.6. Wounds and wound healing

Wounds can be categorised as:
● **Clean** – where the incision is made through uninflamed tissue as part of elective surgery; or surgery where there is no breach in asepsis, e.g. hip replacement, herniorrhaphy.
● **Clean-contaminated** – e.g. emergency surgery; or an elective operation with controlled entry into a visceral tract; or surgery with only a minor breach in aseptic technique, e.g. cholecystectomy.
● **Contaminated** – e.g. penetrating trauma >4 hours; operations with gross spillage from GI tract; or where asepsis is breached, e.g. stab wound.
● **Dirty** – e.g. where there is frank pus; perforation of the GI or urinary tracts, e.g. perforated appendix; or penetrating trauma >4 hours.

Types of wound healing

Wound healing by primary/first intention: describes mechanical closure with direct apposition of the skin edges (e.g. with staples, sutures, glue). This should which ideally be performed <6 hours from time of injury and is the preferred method of wound healing in clean wounds where there is minimal soft tissue loss and healthy tissue. Advantages: results in better cosmesis and healing time compared to healing by secondary intention.

Delayed primary closure: usually performed at day 3–7, in a potentially contaminated wound, with no significant tissue loss, where closure of the wound is preferable.

Healing by secondary intention: heavily contaminated or infected wounds, e.g. abscesses, infected ulcers, are commonly debrided (surgical excision of devitalised tissue and foreign matter, irrigation, vacuum dressing) and allowed to heal in this fashion, which relies on the formation of granulation tissue and contraction. This is a slow process with poor cosmetic results, i.e. prominent scarring.

Factors affecting wound healing

○ **Patient factors:** e.g. malnutrition, malignancy, drugs (e.g. steroids), immobility, obesity, advanced age, smoking, metabolic factors (e.g. jaundice, diabetes, uraemia)
○ **Local factors:** e.g. poor blood supply, wound haematoma +/− infection, contamination/foreign body/infection, poor apposition/necrotic skin edges, wound closure under tension, irradiation to skin

Complications of wounds
- **Immediate:** pain, bleeding.
- **Early:** infection, non-healing, osteomyelitis, sinus/fistula formation.
- **Late:** malignant change, i.e. Marjolin's ulcer, contractures or deformity of adjacent joints, anaemia, heterotrophic calcification, hypertrophic or keloid scar.

21

Critical care

21.1. Shock
Shock is characterised by inadequate organ perfusion resulting in poor tissue oxygenation and failure of removal of toxic metabolites. It can lead to organ failure.

Types of shock

○ Hypovolaemic   ○ Cardiogenic
○ Septic   ○ Anaphylactic
○ Neurogenic

Hypovolaemic shock
Occurs as a result of loss of circulatory volume. Causes: haemorrhage, gastrointestinal loss (using high-output fistulae, vomiting, diarrhoea and third space loss in intestinal obstruction), severe burns, renal loss of water and electrolytes.

CLINICAL FEATURES   Pale, cold, clammy peripheries; a rapid, thready pulse; low blood pressure with postural drop; low urine output; rising creatinine (suggesting inadequate renal perfusion); altered mental state (suggesting poor cerebral perfusion).

MANAGEMENT   Requires resuscitation of the patient (ABC); review of the patient's case notes, observations and drug charts; establishment and treatment of the underlying cause +/− transfer to an HDU/ITU for care +/− referral to a specialist team.
- **Airways:** administer high flow oxygen; assess airway patency.
- **Breathing:** record respiratory rate, oxygen saturations +/− perform ABG; consider respiratory support if inadequate oxygenation or ventilation.
- **Circulation:** record heart rate and BP; establish intravenous access (with two large-bore cannulae); consider central venous line insertion to aid fluid resuscitation; catheterise; perform ECG and send urgent bloods for FBC, U&Es, LFTs, clotting, glucose and cross-match.

Note: resuscitate with intravenous fluid (colloid, saline or Hartmanns) or blood if shock due to haemorrhage.
- **Disability:** AVPU Score (Alert, responsive to Voice, Pain, Unresponsive).
- **Expose:** to identify a cause of shock, e.g. source of bleeding.

Further management may include improvement of end-organ perfusion, e.g. with vasopressor support, and correction of the complications of shock, e.g. acute renal failure, ARDS, coagulopathy.

Cardiogenic shock
Primary cardiac dysfunction – due to myocardial infarction, arrhythmia, dilated cardiomyopathy, acute myocarditis, acute valvular pathology.

Secondary cardiac dysfunction – due to cardiac tamponade, tension pneumothorax, massive pulmonary embolism (PE).

CLINICAL FEATURES   Evidence of poor tissue/end-organ perfusion (as per hypo-volaemic shock above). In addition, there may be evidence of left ventricular failure. An accurate history, examination, ECG and chest x-ray will aid diagnosis. *See Cardiology section* for management.

Septic shock
Circulatory collapse mediated by systemic infection.

CLINICAL FEATURES   In contrast to hypovolaemic or cardiogenic shock, peripheries are typically warm and pink; systemic vascular resistance is reduced (due to vasodilation); pulse may be bounding and the pulse pressure (PP) elevated due to a hyperdynamic circulation (i.e. increased cardiac output). Pyrexia, tachycardia, hypotension are also usually present. *See SIRS, Sepsis and MODS section* for management.

Anaphylactic shock
Systemic, histamine-mediated, allergic reaction, that causes vasodilation of the arterioles and increased capillary permeability resulting in hypotension and loss of fluid/protein into the interstitial space, respectively. Importantly, the airway is at risk from laryngo- and facial oedema in anaphylaxis, and early intubation should be considered in severe cases.

MANAGEMENT   Remove inciting cause. Assess ABC; administer high flow oxygen, fluid resuscitate. If evidence of wheeze, stridor, respiratory distress or shock – give 500 mcg adrenaline IM (repeat in five mins if no improvement), 10 mg IV chlorpheniramine and 100 mg IV hydrocortisone.

Neurogenic shock
An acute loss of peripheral vasomotor tone leading to massive vasodilation and subsequent circulatory collapse. Causes include spinal transection, brainstem injury, deep general anaesthesia and spinal anaesthesia with the block extending to the sympathetic outflow tract.

21.2. Sirs, sepsis and mods
Systemic inflammatory response syndrome (SIRS)
SIRS is the response of the body to an infection or injury (e.g. pancreatitis, burns, multiple trauma and haemorrhagic shock), and is defined by the presence of two or more of the following criteria:
- **Pyrexia** >38° or **hypothermia** <36°.
- **Tachycardia** >90 beats per minute (in the absence of a β-blocker).
- **Tachypnoea** >20 breaths per minute or $PaCO_2$ <4.3kPa.
- **White cell count** >12 or <4 × 10^9/L.

When SIRS occurs in the presence of confirmed infection this is defined as **sepsis**. Major sepsis/septic shock is associated with a high mortality and the most common sites of infection in this group are the chest, abdomen and genitourinary tract.

Multi-organ dysfunction syndrome (MODS)

A dysfunction or failure of two or more systems (i.e. cardiovascular, respiratory, renal, gut, haematological or CNS) due to either the severity of the initial insult or persistence of an activated inflammatory response. Importantly, single-system failure has a mortality of 40%; with three-or-more system failure, mortality approaches 98–100%. Early (within first 6 hours) 'goal directed therapy' is essential to improve survival.

MANAGEMENT

- ABC: high flow oxygen and fluid resuscitation to avoid tissue hypoxia with appropriate monitoring, e.g. urinary catheterisation, CVP line, serial ABGs.
- Septic screen: culture urine, stool, sputum, blood, line tips, drain fluid, wounds.
- Investigations: CXR; ECG (for arrhythmia/ischaemia); blood tests: FBC and clotting (infection, DIC), U&Es (renal failure), LFTs (biliary/pancreatic sepsis), CRP.
- Control of source of sepsis, may involve:
  - **empirical broad spectrum antibiotics** until culture and sensitivity results available
  - **drainage**, e.g. of abscess, empyema, infected haematoma
  - **debridement**, e.g. of infected wounds to reduce bacterial load; necrosectomy
  - **removal of foreign body/device**, e.g. urinary catheter, central or peripheral line, prosthetic graft
  - **definitive surgery**, e.g. amputation in cases of wet or gas gangrene.
- Prevention of complications:
  - DVT prophylaxis
  - nutritional support
  - proton-pump inhibitor (reduces risk of stress ulceration)
  - barrier nursing
  - ensure tight glycaemic control.
- Refer early to ITU/HDU as appropriate.
- Further management may involve: inotropic support; activated protein C (has antithrombotic, anti-inflammatory and profibrinolytic properties), blood products (e.g. plasma, platelets and FFP), haemofiltration/dialysis, chest physiotherapy +/− ventilation.

21.3. Burns

Burns can be classified according to their aetiology, i.e. electrical, thermal, cold or chemical. Factors that will affect outcome include the type, depth and extent of the injury; the age of the patient (with those at the extremes of age performing poorly); the presence of an inhalation injury, and cardio-respiratory disease.

CLINICAL FEATURES

- Evidence of inhalation injury, i.e. soot, carbonaceous sputum, singed facial hair, facial burns, oropharyngeal inflammation, carboxyhaemoglobin >10%.
- Extent of injury can be estimated using *Wallace's 'Rule of Nines'* (*see* Table). *Note*: the palm of the patient's hand corresponds to approximately 1% of the patient's body surface area.

AREA OF BODY	% OF TOTAL BODY SURFACE AREA (BSA)
Head	9%
Anterior aspect of trunk	18%
Posterior aspect of trunk	18%
Arms	9% each
Legs	18% each
Perineum	1%

Depth of thermal burn

○ **First degree** (superficial partial thickness): typically painful and erythematous in appearance. Usually heals within seven days
○ **Second degree** (deep partial thickness): extends into dermis; typically red, painful, blistering and oedematous. Healing occurs without scarring and can take 2–3 weeks
○ **Third degree** (full thickness skin loss): typically painless with a waxy, leathery and charred appearance. Healing occurs with contractures and may require grafting

MANAGEMENT – DETERMINED BY THE TYPE OF INJURY

- ABC: establish and maintain airway early (*Note*: risk of laryngeal oedema with inhalation injuries); consider carbon monoxide poisoning; obtain IV access and fluid resuscitate (*see Parklands formula* as rough rule of thumb).
- Give intravenous opiate analgesia, i.e. morphine, and tetanus prophylaxis.
- Identify and treat associated injuries, i.e. fractures, blunt trauma, blast injury.
- Remove all constrictive clothing and jewellery (due to risk of swelling).
- Prevent hypothermia.
- Insert a nasogastric tube as gastric emptying is often delayed and consider a proton pump inhibitor due to the risk of stress ulceration (Cushing's ulcers).
- Wound care (do not disrupt blisters, use non-adhesive dressings, avoid prophylactic antibiotics).
- Monitor renal function: risk of rhabdomyolysis and myoglobinuria.
- Anaemia may occur in severe burns and necessitate blood transfusion.
- Nutritional support to aid wound healing. Nasogastric rather than parenteral feeding is preferred due to the increased risk of line infection.
- Surgery, e.g. escharotomy or skin grafting.
- Transfer to a burns centre if appropriate.

Parklands formula

Fluid (ml) required in first 24 hours = 4 × weight (kg) × surface area of burn.

Half is given in the first 8 hours, and the remainder over the next 16 hours.

Glossary

AAA	abdominal aortic aneurysm
ABC	airways, breathing and circulation
ABG	arterial blood gas
ACE inhibitor	angiotensin converting enzyme inhibitor
ACE	angiotensin converting enzyme
AChR	acetylcholine receptor
ACL	anterior cruciate ligament
ACS	acute coronary syndromes
ACTH	adrenocorticotropic hormone
AD	Alzheimer's disease
AF	atrial fibrillation
AFB	acid fast bacilli
aka	also known as
ALL	acute lymphoblastic leukaemia
ALP	alkaline phosphatase
AML	acute myeloid leukaemia
ANA	anti-nuclear antibodies
AP	antero-posterior
AR	aortic regurgitation
ARBs	all receptor blockers, e.g. candesartan
ARDS	adult respiratory distress syndrome
AS	aortic stenosis
ASD	atrial septal defect
AVM	arterio-venous malformation
AVN	avascular necrosis
AV node	atrio-ventricular node
AVP	arginine vasopressin
AXR	abdominal x-ray
BCC	basal cell carcinoma
BE	base excess
BM/CBG	capillary blood glucose
BP	blood pressure
CA	coronary artery
Ca^{2+}	calcium
CABG	coronary artery bypass grafting
CBD	common bile duct
CBG	capillary blood glucose
CCF	congestive cardiac failure
CEA	carcinoembryonic antigen
CF	cystic fibrosis
CHB	complete heart block
CIDP	chronic inflammatory demyelinating polyneuropathy

CJD	Creutzfeldt-Jakob disease
CK	creatine kinase
CLL	chronic lymphocytic leukaemia
CML	chronic myeloid leukaemia
CMV	cytomegalovirus
CN	cranial nerves
COPD	chronic obstructive pulmonary disease
CPR	cardio-pulmonary resuscitation
CRF	corticotropin releasing-factor
CSF	cerebrospinal fluid
CT	computed tomography
CTD	connective tissue disorder
CT PA	computed tomography (CT) pulmonary angiogram (PA)
CVA	cerebrovascular accident
CXR	chest x-ray
DC cardioversion	direct current cardioversion
DIP joints	distal interphalangeal joints
DKA	diabetic ketoacidosis
DLB	dementia with Lewy bodies
DM	diastolic murmur
DMARDs	disease-modifying anti-rheumatic drugs
DRE	digital rectal examination
DVT	deep vein thrombosis
EBV	Epstein-Barr virus
ECG	electrocardiogram
EEG	electroencephalogram
ENA	extractable nuclear antigens
EPL	extensor pollicis longus
ERCP	endoscopic retrograde cholangiopancreatogram
ESM	ejection systolic murmur
ESR	erythrocyte sedimentation rate
FAP	familial adenomatous polyposis
FAST	focused assessment with sonography for trauma
FBC	full blood count
FFP	fresh frozen plasma
FNAC	fine needle aspiration for cytology
FOB	faecal occult blood
GA	general anaesthesia
GB	gallbladder
GCS	Glasgow Coma Scale
GGT	gamma-glytamyl transpeptidase
GHRH	growth hormone releasing hormone
GI	gastrointestinal
GnRH	gonadotropin releasing-hormone
GP	general practitioner
HAART	highly active antiretroviral therapy
Hb	haemoglobin
HDCT	heritable disorders of connective tissue
HDU	high dependency unit
HF	heart failure
HI	head injury
HIV	human immunodeficiency virus
HNPCC	hereditary non-polyposis colon cancer

HOCM	hypertrophic obstructive cardiomyopathy
HPA	hypothalamic pituitary axis
HPV	human papillomavirus
HRT	hormone replacement therapy
HS	heart sound(s)
HSV	herpes simplex virus
HT	hypertension
HTLV	human T-cell lymphotropic virus
HUS	haemolytic uraemic syndrome
5-HIAA	5-hydroxyindolacetic acid
IBD	inflammatory bowel disease
IBS	irritable bowel syndrome
ICP	intracranial pressure
ICU	intensive care unit
IE	infective endocarditis
IGF-1	insulin-like growth factor-1
IGT	impaired glucose tolerance
IHD	ischaemic heart disease
IRMAs	intraretinal microvascular abnormalities
IV	intravenous
IVDU	intravenous drug use
IVIg	intravenous immunoglobulin
JVP	jugular venous pressure
K$^+$	potassium
LA	local anaethesia
LBBB	left bundle branch block
LBO	large bowel obstruction
LCL	lateral collateral ligament
LFTs	liver function tests
LIF	left iliac fossa
LOC	loss of consciousness
LMN	lower motor neurone
LP	lumbar puncture
LRTI	lower respiratory tract infection
LUQ	left upper quadrant
LUTS	lower urinary tract symptoms
LVADs	left ventricular assist devices
LVF	left ventricular failure
LVH	left ventricular hypertrophy
MAI	*mycobacterium avium intracellulare*
MCL	medial collateral ligament
MCP	meta-carpophalangeal
MC&S	microscopy, culture and sensitivity
MCTD	mixed connective tissue disease
Mg^{2+}	magnesium
MI	myocardial infarction
MNG	multi-nodular goitre
MODS	multi-organ dysfunction syndrome
MRA	magnetic resonance angiogram
MR	mitral regurgitation
MRI	magnetic resonance imaging
MRV	magnetic resonance venography
MS	multiple sclerosis

MSU	mid-stream urine
MuSK	antibody muscle specific tyrosine kinase
Na$^+$	sodium
NBM	nil by mouth
NCS	nerve conduction studies
NGT	nasogastric tube
NMJ	neuromuscular junction
NOF	neck of femur
NSAIDs	non-steroidal anti-inflammatory drugs
NSTEMI	non-ST elevation MI
OCP	oral contraceptive pill
OGTT	oral glucose tolerance test
OM	otitis media
ORIF	open reduction and internal fixation
OT	occupational therapy/therapist
PCA	patient controlled analgesia
PCI	percutaneous coronary intervention
PCP	pneumocystis pneumonia
PCR	polymerase chain reaction
PCV	packed cell volume
PD	Parkinson's disease
PDA	patent ductus arteriosus
PE	pulmonary embolus
PEFR	peak expiratory flow rate
PI	protease inhibitors
PID	pelvic inflammatory disease
PML	progressive multifocal leucoencephalopathy
PND	paroxysmal nocturnal dyspnoea
PPI	proton pump inhibitor
PPM	permanent pacemaker
PR	per rectal, pulmonary regurgitation
PS	pulmonary stenosis
PSM	pansystolic murmur
PTC	percutaneous transcutaneous cholangiogram
PTCA	percutaneous coronary angioplasty
PTH	parathyroid hormone
PUO	pyrexia of unknown origin
PVD	peripheral vascular disease
RA	rheumatoid arthritis
RAS	renal artery stenosis
RBC	red blood cells
RF	rheumatoid factor
RIF	right iliac fossa
RR	respiratory rate
RSV	respiratory syncytial virus
RTIs	reverse transcriptase inhibitors
RUQ	right upper quadrant
RV	right ventricular
RVF	right ventricular failure
SAH	subarachnoid haemorrhage
SBO	small bowel obstruction
SC	subcutaneous
SCC	squamous cell carcinoma

SIADH	syndrome of inappropriate anti-diuretic hormone secretion
SIRS	systemic inflammatory response syndrome
SLE	systemic lupus erythematosus
SOA	swelling of ankles
SOB	shortness of breath
SOL	space occupying lesion(s)
	swelling of the leg
SVC	superior vena cava
TB	tuberculosis
TCC	transitional cell carcinoma
TEDS	thromboembolic deterrent stockings
TFTs	thyroid function tests
TOE	trans-oesophageal echo
tPA	tissue plasminogen activator
TR	tricuspid regurgitation
TRH	thyrotropin releasing hormone
TSH	thyroxine stimulating hormone
	thyroid stimulating hormone
T3	triiodothyronine
T4	free thyroxine
UC	ulcerative colitis
U&Es	urea and electrolytes
UMN	upper motor neurone
URTI	upper respiratory tract infection
UTI	urinary tract infection
VaD	vascular dementia
VC	vital capacity
VSD	ventricular septal defect
WCC	white cell count
WHO	World Health Organization
WPW	Wolff-Parkinson-White

Index